Here's what others are saying about *Feeling Great At 88* by Dick Brown:

"There are many qualities of Richard Brown's life-style that surely are a part of God's grace enabling him to still 'feel great at eighty-eight,' but I single out two: his 'excellent spirit' (Dan. 6:3), and his regular exercise program that includes golf and even tennis! And of course his stable and happy home-life with his wife has played a key role also."

- Daniel P. Fuller, son and only child of Charles and Grace Fuller; former President of Gospel Broadcasting Association and Fuller Evangelistic Association

"In these pages, the author testifies that he sees himself as 'a radio that is tuned in to God's voice.' The signal is very clear in this warm and inspiring book. Dick Brown broadcasts much wisdom about the kind of abundant living that gets us ready for eternity!"

- Richard J. Mouw, President and Professor of Christian Philosophy, Fuller Theological Seminary

"Why does Dick Brown have more energy at 88 than I do at 38? Because Dick has intentionally implemented a biblical, comprehensive plan for his health. His years of experience offer a wealth of wisdom to generations young and old."

- Chad Zaucha, Senior Pastor of First Baptist Church, Ojai, California

"Uniquely, this inspirational book blends autobiography with sage advice on achieving a healthy, balanced life. From one who knows—an 88 year-old pastor, quartet baritone, and World War II Seabee; comes the wisdom of age and common sense mingled with Christian devotion nurtured over eight decades since his conversion at age 9. It's a rewarding treasury of day-to-day miscellanies, from named food supplements to exercise to tithing to weathering the storms of pain personally and in the family. All from the patriarchal voice of one with a loving spouse, nine children, 32 grandchildren, and 20 great grandchildren."

- Russ Spittler, Provost Emeritus and Professor of New Testament Emeritus, Fuller Seminary, Pasadena, California

"To live by medicine is to live horribly. In an age where government is attempting to steal our health care system and fewer and fewer people are willing to take any responsibility for their own life and health, Dick Brown offers a wonderfully uplifting alternative to aging, illness and decrepitude."

- John Galt, author of *Dreams Come Due*

"Wisdom is woven into the heart of this book... whether you're 28, 58 or 88, you'll find ideas, insights and inspiration to be all that God intended you to be."

- Susan Whitcomb, author and Christian career/life coach, Founder/President of the Academies

FEELING GREAT AT 88

By
Richard Ewing Brown, Jr.
with Matthew Kinne

FEELING GREAT AT 88

Published by:
Intermedia Publishing Group, Inc.
P.O. Box 2825
Peoria, Arizona 85380
www.intermediapub.com

ISBN 978-1-935529-48-4

Printed in the United States of America
by Epic Print Solutions

Acknowledgements

First, I must thank the God of the Bible for giving me great health for these 88 years. This book would not have been possible without Your Presence in my life.

Next, I'd like to recognize these friends and champions who have contributed to the great health I now enjoy today: my parents: Richard Ewing Brown, Sr. and Greta Marie Johnson Brown; my siblings: Helen Etheleen Brown Fiske, Harsh Jay Brown, George Douglas Brown; my friends: Charles E. Fuller, M. Howard Fagan, James Earl Ladd, Coach Hamilton, Coach Elder, Eloise Sill Sullivan, Barbara M. Brown, Carl and Sybil Kessler, Karl Irvin, Jr., Chuck Swindoll, James Dobson, Art Waters, Jack Coleman, Harry and Margaret Riley, Sam Smith, Gary Wells, Bill MacDougall, Warren Smith, Art Jaissle, Rudy Atwood, Stanley Lindquist, Faculty/Students at Schools of Learning, and members of Churches where I've served.

Next, I'd like to recognize the fine writing abilities of my collaborator, Matthew Kinne. Your organization, skills and talent are superb! And, I'd like to thank Terry Whalin and everyone at Intermedia Publishing for your leadership and publishing expertise.

Last, I'd like to thank my beloved wife, Margaret Ann Brown, and our wonderful combined families.

Many more of you have made a significant impact on my life. I apologize for not mentioning your names. I am very grateful to you all for helping me to be who and what I am today! Richard Ewing Brown, Jr.

Dedication

This book is dedicated to the three greatest loves of my life: God the Father, God the Son, and God the Holy Spirit; and to, humanly speaking, the greatest love of my life over the past 36 years, my beloved wife, confidante, companion, best friend, sweetheart, encourager, and constructive critic, who, Praise God, took seriously and literally her promise on June 16, 1973 in Manteca, California to stick by me "for better or for worse." I love you, Margaret Ann Brown.

Richard Ewing Brown, Jr., Ojai, California

My God and I

My God and I, go in the field together
We walk and talk as good friends should and do,
We clasp our hands, our voices ring with laughter,
My God and I, walk through the meadows hue.
We clasp our hands, our voices ring with laughter
My God and I, walk through the meadows hue.

He tells me of the years that went before me.
When heav'nly plans were made for me to be,
When all was but a dream of dim conception,
To come to life, earth's verdant glory see
When all was but a dream of dim conception,
To come to life earth's verdant glory see.

My God and I, will go for aye together,
We'll walk and talk and jest as good friends do,
This earth will pass and with it common trifles,
But God and I, will go unendingly.
This earth will pass and with it common trifles,
But God and I will go unendingly.

As I'll approach the portal high,
Then shall the voice of the watchman cry;
"Enter, O tired ones, saved by His grace!"
I shall look up and see His face.
We'll clasp our hands, Our Voices ring with laughter,
My God and I will go unendingly.

- J.B. Sergei and A.A. Wihtol, ©1935

Foreword

Having spent 34 years in the military and rising to the rank of Lieutenant General, I have often been asked which leader had the biggest influence on my life. Without hesitation I have always answered my dad, Dick Brown. It truly took becoming a grown man myself and even a father to realize the impact my dad did, in fact, have on my life. But from my earliest memories to the present my dad was steady and faithful to his integrity, moral conviction, and faith in the living God and his son Jesus Christ. He absolutely practiced what he preached and yes, he even preaches a little in this book. What would you expect from a Preacher!

This book gives a glimpse to the life he has lived and is a compilation of his stories and living testimony. He highlights his beliefs, his practices, and his steadfastness to keeping in shape physically and spiritually. He gives the reader practical applications of how and when to do those things that will make you feel "Great" into your later years. Although it is never too late to start, the younger you start putting these principles into practice the better your opportunity of living a longer, more fruitful life on earth as well as enjoying eternity with our Lord.

Dad shares his secrets with his audience and I can attest to his superb physical, emotional, mental and spiritual shape at the age of 88. To this day he walks two miles a day, plays tennis and golf every week and has to find competitors well under his age to have a real game. He is close to shooting his age in golf and might have done it already if he would just move forward to the senior tees! He is a man who has certainly suffered setbacks in his life, but through even those he has taught me great lessons in the power of faith and the value of seeing the good in everything and everyone. His standard answer to my regular query of: "So Pop, how you doing today?" is usually; "Why it's the best day of my life!" And for him each day is a wonderful gift from God; to be filled with things done for the glory of God.

He has something to say about life, faith, and truth. You will be glad you read his lessons and stories and when finished you will see he has lived Joshua 24:15, "As for me and my household, we will serve the Lord."

U.S. Air Force Lieutenant General (Retired)
Richard "Tex" Ewing Brown III

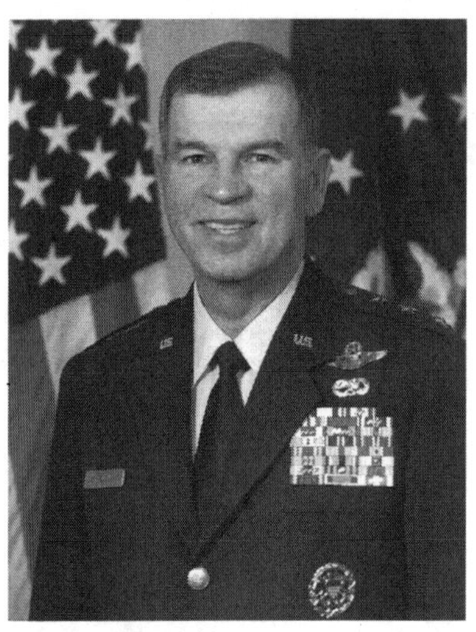

DISCLAIMER

The words in this book are solely the opinion of the author, Richard E. Brown, Jr. Mr. Brown is not a health specialist, medical doctor or health professional. As such, *Feeling Great at 88* includes no health guarantees and is not meant to diagnose, cure or prevent any adverse health conditions. Consult with your doctor or health specialist before beginning any new health regimen.

Table of Contents

Living Your Great Health

What Is Great Health?

Introduction
The Reason for the Hope I Have

Then we will no longer be infants, tossed back and forth by the waves, and blown here and there by every wind of teaching and by the cunning and craftiness of men in their deceitful scheming. Instead, speaking the truth in love, we will in all things grow up into Him who is the Head, that is, Christ. From Him the whole body, joined and held together by every supporting ligament, grows and builds itself up in love, as each part does its work. - Ephesians 4:14-16

But in your hearts set apart Christ as Lord. Always be prepared to give an answer to everyone who asks you to give the reason for the hope that you have. But do this with gentleness and respect. -1 Peter 3:15

I am 88 years of age and I am feeling great. Spiritually, physically, mentally and emotionally, I'm enjoying excellent health! Would you like to know why? If so, please read on!

I have a passion for great health. The reason for my passion is personal, but I believe you can have great health, too! I am not a physician, nor do I have an advanced degree in medicine, nutrition, physiology or health. What I do have is a life touched by the grace and mercy of God. This book is basically a testimony, a biography of God's grace, mercy and instruction into my life, and a record of the health choices that I have made in response to His leading. I am who I am today solely because of God's presence in my life.

As you age into your senior years, your path to great health may involve different exercises, foods and strategies than mine. I only know what has worked for me, a retired pastor with a vast, rich life filled with great health (and a few health scares too). Nevertheless, I hope that my lifestyle choices will work for you, too, and give you great health no matter your age or circumstance in life.

There is a reason for the hope I enjoy. I believe that the foundations of great health lie in believing in and obeying the God of the Bible. Many Christians do not enjoy excellent health, physically speaking. Their mouths praise God but their waist lines bow to a different ruler. These believers may enjoy excellent spiritual, emotional, mental and moral health, but they ignore the fact that their body is the "temple of the Holy Spirit" (1 Cor. 6:19). Good overall health begins and is sustained by a solid spiritual foundation. Nevertheless, a strong spiritual foundation doesn't guarantee that every aspect of health will fall in line. Being a strong and devout Christian does not guarantee excellent physical health.

Irregardless of where you are spiritually, whether you are one of the strongest Christian believers or one of the most hardened staunch atheists, my argument for good health starts with and is sustained by an accurate, dynamic faith in the God of the Bible. It is here where healthy personal stewardship grows and is practiced.

My daily choices, behaviors and subsequent lifestyle stem from this foundation. It's difficult to rate which of these choices are more important than the other because their effects on my health are cumulative and interrelated. If I would have to rate these things on a scale of one to ten, everything would deserve a ten. I do so many different things contributing to my great health. For now, here is just a taste of some of the things I do and believe that are important to me. In later chapters, I'll explore how and why these and other things work for me and suggest how they could work for you, too.

Spiritually, I attend church regularly, trust constantly in the Father, Son and Holy Spirit, pray often, read my Bible daily, plus look at the insights of five Christian believers found in five separate written daily devotionals. I confess my sins and receive forgiveness. I write a tithe and offering check each week and fellowship with other Christians. I converse with non-Christians and share with them the hope I have in Christ.

I perform my daily calisthenics, take daily walks, and play golf and tennis. I sleep nine to ten hours every 24 hours (including nap time), and stick with a daily routine.

My faith informs my diet. Daily, I eat sensibly: I eat half an apple per day, take some eight food supplements each morning, and I drink lots of water each day, especially in the morning and even in the middle of the night when I get up to relieve myself. I believe all of these factors contribute to the fact that I also have great bowel movements, which is an essential component to maintaining great health.

For my mental and emotional health, I strive daily to

maintain a positive attitude. I sing out loud and in my heart, and I have fantastic loving experiences with my beloved wife such as taking walks on the beaches of the Pacific Ocean and watching beautiful sunrises and sunsets. I learn to say "no" and to say "yes." I write rambling thoughts such as these, do good deeds, and laugh a lot.

Can you see how many of these activities overlap as they relate to the different elements of great health? If I take a walk with my wife on the beach, I'm helping my physical, emotional and mental health. If I eat a wholesome meal with my family, I'm helping the same three elements of health. And if I pray before this meal and/or fellowship with my family about the goodness of God, I benefit from all four aspects of health: spiritual, physical, mental and emotional. Great health is a lifestyle, and the sooner you accept this lifestyle, the better off you'll be. You can't predict how many years you'll have in your life, but you can help control the quality of life in your years. So please join me on this journey. Keep reading about the comprehensive great health I enjoy! (And you can too!)

Chapter 1
Called to Live A Healthy Life

Godliness has value for all things, holding promise for both the present life and the life to come. - 1 Timothy 4:8

Therefore come out from them and be separate, says the Lord. Touch no unclean thing, and I will receive you. - 2 Corinthians 6:17

I believe great health is largely a choice. We often cannot help the evil that strikes us, but our lifestyle choices will add up and greatly contribute to either a victorious life of great health or a life of constant health struggles and even sorrow. We can choose to be a non-smoker and avoid alcoholic beverages. We can choose to consume fewer calories and eat more healthy foods. We can choose to exercise. We can choose to praise God, go to church and serve our community. We can choose to be happy, even when adversity strikes. How you choose to react to unfortunate events will significantly affect your mental, emotional, spiritual, and physical health. To a large extent, you can control your health destiny.

If I had to choose one quote from all the writings of the world to serve as my guidepost for the great health I enjoy,

I believe I would choose Philippians 4: 4 from the Bible: "Rejoice in the Lord always!! I will say it again: Rejoice!!" (Two exclamation points are added for double emphasis.) Rejoicing in the Lord, the God of the Bible, has contributed more to my great health than I could ever have imagined.

First, the word "Rejoice" is telling me to *be positive.* When I count my blessings and give thanks in all things, I'm saying to my body and emotions, I want to feel great. I say to myself, "I'm going to live victoriously, regardless of my circumstances." It's not just a matter of mind-over-matter; it's a command for my body to line up with the blessings that God has promised me in His Word.

Second, by rejoicing in the Lord, I'm reminding myself Who and where my help comes from. I'm not psyching myself out with good thoughts. I'm evoking blessing from the one Living God Who alone can give me great health.

Our Precious Lord created me and gave me breath. Without Him I am like a piece of inanimate clay, lifeless. With Him I am animate and have life. So, whatever happens to me, good times and bad times, sickness and health, through the tough situations and the good moments, etc., I have learned to "rejoice in the Lord always" and, as He has promised, He has rewarded me.

A Biblical Foundation for Health

Hebrews 11:6 says, "And without faith it is impossible to please God, because anyone who comes to Him must believe that He exists and that He rewards those who earnestly seek Him." In March, 1931, I put my faith in the God of the Bible. Since then, I have earnestly sought Him, known Him, loved

Him, served Him, and carried out His assignments for me with the strength that He has given me. While God is my protector (Ps. 32:7), healer (Exod. 15:26) and an "ever present help in times of trouble" (Ps. 46:1), my first assignment is to take care of the most precious gift he has given me: my body. If I don't take care of my body, I insult God and I hinder the work and purposes He has for me in the world. I deny myself the opportunity for God to use me and bless me in the world. When my body is functioning well, I can carry out all of the other assignments He has given me with the best chance for success.

It is my pleasure and honor to take care of the body and mind God has given me because I realize it is through my body and mind that I can experience all that life has to offer. My body and mind are precious.

Some of the most astounding and sometimes hard to believe statements in the entire Bible are about the human body and mind.

- "Don't you know that you yourselves are God's temple and that God's Spirit lives in you? If anyone destroy God's temple, God will destroy him; for God's temple is sacred and you are that temple." (1 Cor. 3:16-17)

- "He who unites himself with the Lord is one with Him in Spirit. Flee from sexual immorality. All other sins a man commits are outside his body but he who sins sexually sins against his own body.

> Do you not know that your body is a temple of the Holy Spirit Who is in you, Whom you have received from God? You are not your own, you were bought at a price. Therefore honor God with your body." (1 Cor. 6:17-20)

If you ever hear somebody joking and saying, "My body is a temple," don't laugh. It's true! This flesh, blood, brains and systems that add up to life are the stuff God made. It is through this stuff that He "lives and moves and has His being" (Acts 17:28).

Another important scripture that speaks to me is Psalm 139. It says my body is fearfully and wonderfully made. My organs, systems and functions were not the result of millions of years of chance occurrences (evolution) but by the brilliant plans of a master designer. The more science advances into the future, the more detail is revealed about our bodies indicating a genius Creator.

Respect for the Body God has Given Me

I love, respect and appreciate my body. Does that sound prideful or arrogant? It shouldn't. I think you should love, respect and appreciate your body, too. It's the only one you have and it is God's gift to you. It is mind boggling to me when I stop and think, daily, that this body in which I've lived for 88-plus years is the temple of the Holy Spirit. It really doesn't belong to me. It is "on loan" to me from my Creator, and He is using my body as one of His homes for Himself, His Son and His Holy Spirit. This may sound crazy to you, but this astounding truth is also found in John 14, where Jesus elaborates on the Blessed Trinity coming to this planet and establishing homes *inside* the bodies of all true Christian believers.

The more I recognize and believe in the profound truths God says about my body, the more I invariably desire to practice faithful stewardship over the use and care of my body. Not only did God create me, He purchased me for His use by Jesus Himself on the Cross. There, He paid the penalty for my sins. (Many non-believers find it difficult to accept the blood sacrifice that God did on our behalf. How I praise and thank God I don't have to understand, I just have to believe it.)

My respect for my body (and all human bodies) began at an early age.

The Defining Moment of my Youth

I was born January 28, 1922 in San Dimas, California, Los Angeles County. My father was the Pastor of First Christian Church, part of Disciples of Christ, not a denomination at that time but part of what was known as "The Restoration Movement" whose goal was to restore New Testament Christianity and the unity of Christ's Church here on earth. My father earned his B.A. from Johnson Bible College in Johnson City, Tennessee, near Knoxville and started graduate school at Drake University in Des Moines, Iowa, where he met and married my mother, Greta Marie Johnson, from Alhambra, California. The first World War cut off my father's education at Drake so he enlisted in the U.S. Navy Chaplain Corps, resigning his commission at war's end and then began to pastor in Clarion, Iowa.

My father became the pastor of First Christian Church, in Merced, California in 1923 and then the pastor of First Christian Church, in Dinuba, California in 1926. He remained at this position until December, 1934 when he passed away at age 41 of leukemia. Medical doctors were unable to decide the nature of his illness until after his passing.

My father took his ministry so very seriously that he did not properly care for his body and physical needs. He would take very short naps when he tired in order to get all the work done that was expected. For a dedicated pastor, a five-minute nap was quite common in the afternoon. Damage to the bone marrow, the accumulation of immature white blood cells, and the onset of anemia eventually took over his body. My father was unable to fight off the ravages of leukemia.

His untimely and early passing had a profound effect on me. I began to think about mortality and health. As I matured towards adulthood and even to this day, I thought about what I could do and how I could think and act to best preserve the health God had given me. I didn't want to die young like my father. My convictions and overall approach to daily living is still informed and overshadowed by the memories and health practices (or lack thereof) practiced by my father.

The Aftermath of his Death

At the time of my father's passing, my sister, Helen Etheleen Brown, was 14, I was 12, my brother, Harsh Jay Brown was 10, and my youngest brother, George Douglas Brown, was 8. Our entire family was devastated. Our father was a very popular figure in our small town of Dinuba and much loved by 200 church members. An influential elder in the church had been able to keep our father out of the Christian Church Pension Fund, saying God would take care of His servants. So, because we had nowhere else to go, my family continued to live in a parsonage next door to the church for a brief time.

Our family had very little cash and so our church members, many of them farming people, met many of the food needs of our family. Hand-me-down clothes were always appreciated and the entire family benefited from the generosity of such church members. These acts of kindness taught me the value of generosity and community – values I still practice today – values that still contribute to my great health.

The only life insurance my father had was a $10,000 Life Insurance Policy with the Veterans' Administration from his World War One days. It proved to be a life-saver and my family was able to make a down payment on three acres of land outside Dinuba with a huge farmhouse and a nice barn. Several family members and friends told me that I was now the *man* of the family and this responsibility weighed heavily on my mind, heart, soul, and body. Although the stress of this responsibility was burdensome, it taught me the value of taking care of what's yours. If I was a carefree kid without responsibility, I may not have readily learned discipline and stewardship. I worked our land as my family tried to make ends meet on our three little acres with two milk cows, many laying hens and frying chickens, a big vegetable garden, and several fruit trees, etc.

As the months and years passed since my father died, I decided to take great strides in taking care of my body. Even at a young age, because I had heard and believed my father's teaching, I understood my body to be the temple of the Holy Spirit. I believed then and I still believe today that God the Father/Son/Holy Spirit actually live inside my body – working out Their good pleasure in me to bless me and others through me.

A Healthy Young Man

After my father died, my mother went to work for the Federal Government making calls on the needy in our area, i.e. those who needed financial help. Her heart for the poor became an example to me of Christian charity and compassion. I realized from her that good emotional, spiritual, physical, and mental health demanded thinking about and doing good for others.

So, my outgoing personality and my emerging heart for other people (as nurtured by my mother) led me to school politics. I finished my first year of high school in Dinuba and was elected President of the Freshman Class. Throughout high school, I performed odd jobs around the community to help make ends meet. These odd jobs also got me out into the community, where I learned to share and relate well with others. At the same time, my mother decided she was being called back into Christian Ministry.

She decided she needed more education, since she had previously dropped out of Drake University after only two years of education there. This act of courage further reinforced in my mind the importance of education and taking care of my mental health. Mom sent Etheleen to Chapman College (then in Hollywood, now Chapman University in Orange, California), and she sent me to Three Rivers, California to live with her sister and family,

Don and Merle Raybourn and their son Bob. Bob was my cousin, only six months my junior.

This transition was difficult because I still attended school in Woodlake. I spent my sophomore year at Woodlake High School, riding the school bus every school day from Three Rivers to Woodlake, a distance of 80 miles roundtrip. Even so, the football, basketball, and baseball coaches at Woodlake took a liking to me and gave me great encouragement to play these sports. I joined all three teams and performed quite well at all of them. This paved the way for me to reach for the goal of becoming an athletic coach and school teacher. It also paved the way to me eventually receiving an athletic scholarship at Chapman College in September of 1939.

I Sing Because I'm Happy

Back to 1937, my mother was offered the position of Associate Pastor of the First Christian Church of Santa Ana, California in Orange County and was able to pull the family back together again. This gave us all a boost for our emotional well-being. After my successful sophomore year at Woodlake, I had two great years at Santa Ana High School and excelled in football, basketball, and baseball. I played tennis for fun but was not on the school team because as the man of the family, I had several odd jobs around Santa Ana and I turned the money over to my mother to help with living expenses.

Then, I received an athletic scholarship offer to Chapman. This was a godsend since my family was always short of cash. My sister was doing well at Chapman and she was the very accomplished school pianist, much loved and appreciated by faculty and students. She was a senior when I arrived as a freshman and she let it be known that I was her younger brother. I had taken voice lessons in Santa Ana when a local and prominent voice teacher took a liking to me and offered me voice lessons in exchange for keeping his studio clean and keeping his yard at home looking nice. To me, this was a great deal.

My sister let it be known that I could not only sing but I was also good at reading music. The Cardinal Quartet at Chapman was the #1 Public Relations Group for the college and had a tremendous reputation all over California, North and South. The first Cardinal Quartet in the early 1930s decided to stay together and became The King's Men, the leading male quartet in Hollywood, landing many jobs, including the *Fibber McGhee and Molly* show. The Cardinal Quartet, at the time of my arrival, was the #3 Quartet at Chapman and, unbeknownst to me, they needed a baritone. My sister urged me to audition but I hesitated, saying they were way out of my class. However, at her urging, I auditioned and was thrilled, of course, to be singing with such "professionals." My abilities could be described as passable, but I was not surprised when the leader of the group said I was too young and inexperienced. Only 17 years old, he said my voice lacked maturity.

I wrote the experience off as a great but fleeting opportunity. I would have better luck next time, with something else. Three weeks later, I was literally shocked, amazed and astounded when I received a small notice in my college mailbox that simply said: You have been selected to sing in the Chapman College Cardinal Quartet. I couldn't believe it and immediately I contacted my sister to find out what was going on. It turns out she spoke to the Head of the Music Department, who was the final authority over the Quartet but had previously stayed in the background on important decisions. Yet, after listening to Etheleen, he decided to start from scratch and picked the members of the Quartet himself. I was chosen as baritone!

The leader who said that I was too young was ousted. A fine second tenor, Art Waters, who had transferred to Chapman from Northwest Christian College in Eugene, Oregon, was in. Art would eventually become my best friend and mentor, taking the place of my father since he was ten years older and quite mature. The importance of being in the Quartet cannot be overstated since the College paid for my room, board, tuition, and traveling expenses. I gave up my athletic scholarship so another athlete could benefit, but I continued with the athletic programs at Chapman, sustained by the singing money instead of the scholarship.

The four years with the Quartet proved to be great preparation for my years with perhaps the best-known Gospel Quartet in the world, Charles E. Fuller's Old Fashioned Revival Hour Quartet, which sang live every Sunday afternoon at the Municipal Auditorium in Long Beach, California. This quartet also sang at the Country Church of Hollywood and was also known as the Goose Creek Quartet.

I thought I was destined for a life in coaching and athletics, but God had other plans. My singing voice, which I developed with disciplined effort, became my calling card and my eventual meal ticket at school. By perfecting my talent, singing with others, and sharing the gospel through song at the same time, I was able to take care of all aspects of my health. Yet one passion of mind still demanded attention.

My Political Passions

In the 7th grade, I lost being elected President of the Student Body by one vote. This failure rattled my self-esteem, but I was encouraged by friends to run again in 8th grade. I, however, instead satisfied myself to successfully run for a position called Head of Recreation Equipment. With that election, I gained my first political victory.

Then in my first year of High School at Dinuba High, my friends nominated me for Class President and I won. My next adventure into "politics" was my first year at Chapman College. To my surprise, at the first meeting of our Freshman Class, I was outright, without warning, elected Class President. To this day, I still don't know how that happened because I didn't run for the office or even show any interest in the position. It just happened, and the event gave me a great big boost causing my self-confidence to soar. Three years later, I ran for President of the entire Student Body and I was elected!

As a Freshmen President, I knew I would one day be "kidnapped." This treasured tradition at Chapman happened to all Freshman Presidents and I knew that it would happen sooner or later to me. My survival ability was stretched, but my wits and great health were up for the challenge. I taped some quarters to the soles of my feet since I knew the sophomores would one day lift my wallet, watch, belt, some of my clothes, shoes, etc. So one night on my way to the library, about ten sophomores jumped me and I was simply overpowered.

They blindfolded me, tied my hands and feet, put me in a car and away we went, driving for about three hours. When the car stopped, one of them said we were on the estate of John Barrymore, the famous actor. They pushed me out of the car and I was left alone under a full moon with many stars and planets shining brightly. I crawled under the tractor and tried to get a little sleep. At sunrise, I could see Barrymore's mansion in the distance and a caretaker's house nearby. I chose to walk to the caretaker's house, and was warmly received by a Hispanic family, and fed breakfast. The head of the family said he was going into Los Angeles and would take me with him. We drove to L.A. and he dropped me off downtown, I took off my socks, got my quarters, found a pay phone, and called my Quartet buddy who came into L.A. to pick me up.

At Chapman, I changed my major to Business Administration and I loved the courses in that program. At the time, Chapman just entered into an agreement with the Navy for the Navy to take over our Hollywood campus. The student body would merge onto the campus of Whittier College in Whittier, California for an indefinite period of time. This unsettled me, and I began to feel the urge to transfer to Occidental College in Pasadena, California, thinking Occidental was better known in educational fields and my chances of getting a coaching/teaching job would increase.

I let my thoughts be known on campus, but several of my classmates strongly encouraged me to continue my stay at Chapman (on the Whittier campus). In spite of my discouraging remarks, they nominated me for Student Body President. I protested, saying I might be transferring, but they were persistent. I won the election handily and was so overwhelmed by their support that I decided I would stick with Chapman. Whittier College had a Quaker background. A fine school, President-to-be Richard Nixon was Student Body President there seven years earlier. I had a great experience at Whittier, and in retrospect, I'm so glad I stayed.

I asked the President of Chapman if he would pay my room, board, and tuition if I put together a new Cardinal Quartet and continue doing promotional work for the college. He enthusiastically said "Yes!" I ended up getting my college degree and later my Master of Divinity without owing a dime – one of the most financially healthy decisions I ever made.

Look Back and Look Ahead

By the end of my college years, I had firmly begun to establish life-long patterns for living a life of great health. My childhood experiences, both planned and unplanned, shaped and modeled me to be the kind of person I am today. Even if you make deliberate health choices today that are contrary to how you behaved as a child, your young life is what you measure your current life against.

Obviously, you can't change the past, but you can change how you both feel about the past and what you will now do with the information you learned in the past. You can forgive others for hurts done against you, deliberate or not. You can pick up some of the good habits of those around you who made wise health decisions, or you can conscientiously choose to act, live, think and eat differently from those you know who have made poor health decisions.

Look back on this chapter and see how I responded to the events of my life. Look back on your own life and see where other people and events helped shape your attitudes of health. Look back and realize what choices you made that contribute to the level of great health you do or do not enjoy today. Once you understand what happened to you, and what you have decided to do about it, you can begin to make deliberate choices today that will contribute to the best health you can have for the rest of your life.

In chapters to come, you'll learn more about my life, my Navy years, my first marriage, and my professional and personal life. I'll relate more and more stories of how God has given me the choice to choose things that will give me great health or choices that will lead to poor health. In the next chapter, I'll explore the four layers of health, what they are, and what is the most foundational layer of them all – an essential ingredient of great health for anyone.

Chapter 2
The Four Layers of Good Health

Who is it He is trying to teach? To whom is He explaining His message? To children weaned from their milk, to those just taken from the breast? For it is: Do and do, do and do, rule on rule, rule on rule, a little here, a little there.

- Isaiah 28: 9-11

Perseverance must finish its work so that you may be mature and complete, not lacking anything.

- James 1:4

A popular device in pop psychology today is to describe essential tenants of good health by using the term "pillars" – you know, those long, tall columns usually made of marble. The program, "Character Counts!" lists the *six* pillars of character: trustworthiness, respect, responsibility, fairness, caring, and citizenship.[1] Another example is Don Colbert's book *The Seven Pillars of Health.* He lists seven pillars to good health, all focusing on food and exercise. Although pillars may be tall, strong and supportive, they have their limitations. What help are they when the *foundations* of health are threatened? It's time for a new model for health.

Look at the following figures. In **Figure 1**, notice how thin the four pillars are. Notice how tall they are versus how narrow their base is. In fact, the taller the pillars become, the more unstable the structure becomes.

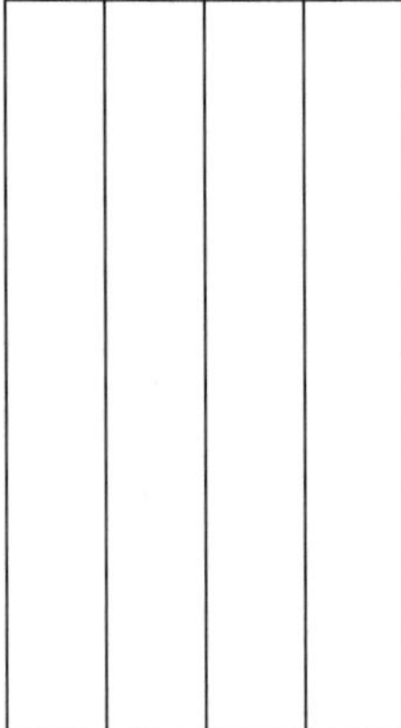

Figure 1. – Four Thin, Tall Pillars

Now look at **Figure 2**. Notice how thick the four layers are. Notice how wide they are versus how narrow their base is. If the layers widen further, the structure only becomes stronger. It's time for layers to replace pillars as the new model of health.

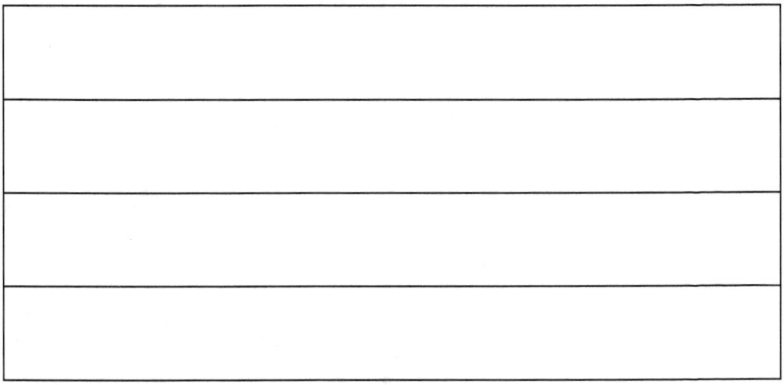

Figure 2. – Four Fat, Wide Layers

One of my favorite bible verses is Matthew 7:25. It reads, "The rain came down, the streams rose, and the winds blew and beat against that house; yet it did not fall, because it had its foundation on the rock." The difference between a standing house and a house swept away is not its pillars, but its foundation. Pillars are insufficient against the strong winds and rains of life. It's the foundation that matters. The foundations in my life have given me a great difference in my overall health. They are the reason I have enjoyed great health my whole life.

The Bible verses Mathew 7:26 and 27 continue to tell of the importance of foundations. They are a warning worth heeding: "But everyone who hears these words of Mine and does not put them into practice is like a foolish man who built his house on sand. The rain came down, the streams rose, and the winds blew and beat against that house, and it fell with a great crash."

I don't want to fall with a crash and I don't want you to fall with a crash of any kind, at all. I want you to stand upright with me when the storms of life hit. If they haven't hit you already, beware! They will. But you can weather the storms with a solid foundation. Pillars can blow over in a strong wind or topple over when their base is eroded. Layers, however, create a firm foundation, which are much harder to move because the weight isn't resting on a small area, but over a broad base. Layers have the *full*, *entire* support of the substance they are lying against.

Jesus speaks about laying a foundation on a solid rock. The rock to which Jesus is referring to is Himself. It is this same rock where I lay my foundation. I believe the basis for good health, or the ground level foundation for good health, must be a strong spirituality based on worshipping and obeying the God of the Bible. Worshipping and obeying a god other than the God of the Bible, (such as yourself, your career, money, success, pleasure, or any of the other world religions) may give you some order and meaning, but ultimately it will end in ruin because at best, false religions are sincere but misguided. Ultimately, all false religions are based on lies, and will lead to death, destruction, ruin, and sadly, eternal separation from God – the ultimate in poor eternal health.

Thankfully, a vibrant spirituality based on the God of the Bible will lay the platform for the other layers of great health to rest. When you are a believing, worshipping, and obedient Christian, operating out of joy, humility and gratitude to the God of the Bible, your ability to obtain physical health will be optimum. No longer will your reasons for physical health be trite and/or fleeting, such as "I want to look great in a swimsuit." No. Your reasons for taking care of yourself physically are deeper, richer, and more valuable. You want to be the best you that you can be because you see the value you are in God's eyes. You see yourself for loving and being loved, serving and being served, and honoring and obeying God to be the best you can be for Christ and His Kingdom.

When your heart and life are right before the God of the Bible and your physical life (good eating and good exercise) is laid down on top of that, you position your mental and emotional health to act and react with optimal performance, too. Some mental and emotional issues stem from poor eating or abuse of the body (such as drug use). Lethargy and laziness can result in depression – a physical health issue with a large emotional health component. But a sharp mind is one that has purpose and a correct balance of electrolytes for optimal performance. All the neural synapses are firing quickly and efficiently. This person also laughs, loves, and cries appropriately – being emotional but not reacting in any way inappropriate to the stimuli around him. This person is a complete, whole person.

Let's look at a third figure which represents the four layers of great health – **Figure 3**.

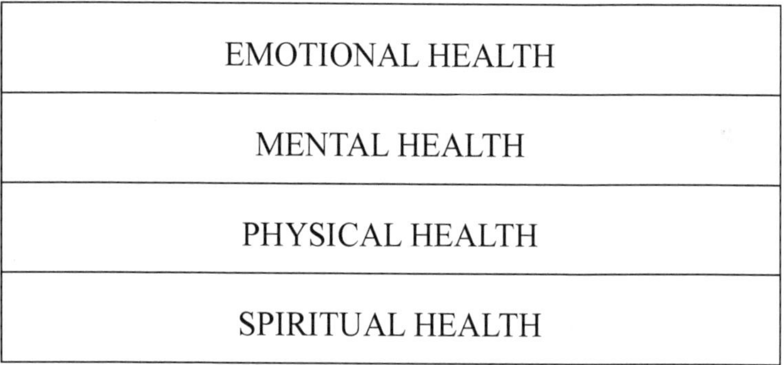

Figure 3. – The Four Layers of Health

A person with a vibrant spirituality based on worshipping and obeying the God of the Bible (great spiritual health), taking care of his physical body (great physical health), using his sharp mind (great mental health) to relate well with others and reacting well to events good and bad (great emotional health) are what define great health. It is this cumulative, dynamic layering of health that allows me to feel great at 88.

To further understand the different layers of health we all have, and to discover how I have lived them, keep reading below. I'll describe what these layers mean to me and I'll include stories from my past on how these layers have worked out in my daily life. These and many other testimonies of God's goodness throughout my life have made it easier for me to make better, healthier choices. God's goodness is why I now enjoy great health well into my senior years. I feel great at 88 because God has led me successfully through many health traps. Come and learn about the goodness of God, and how great health can be true for you, too.

The Spiritual Health Layer

I believe a firm spiritual foundation is absolutely essential for great health. Every health choice you (and I) make comes from the spiritual worldview we individually hold. If you don't value human life very much because you don't see yourself created (as Gen. 1:27 says) "in the image of God," then you'll make poor health choices. If you believe you are a redeemed, child of God, made by God, for God, and filled with God's Spirit, then you're more likely to take care of the temple (body) He has given you. The most spiritually healthy choice I ever made was the choice to accept Jesus Christ as my Lord and Savior when I was 9. Since that moment, when God gave me new life, He has daily revealed Himself to me, always leading me to relinquish control of my life to Him. Simply said, the Holy Spirit now guides me to make healthy lifestyle choices.

As a sinner saved by Grace, I haven't always followed God's leading in my life, but when I gain some direction from His Word (the Bible) and/or hear His voice in my heart, I strive to obey. The result or "fruit" of obeying Him becomes clearly evident – a closer fellowship with God, and ultimately better health.

When I became a Christian, God entered my life and began to lead and guide me. This has been a wonderful, marvelous way of living because it gets me out of the way. Instead of having to wrack my brain for answers to life's dilemmas, I simply lean on God and He gives me understanding for what I'm lacking. In fact, throughout my life, God has gotten me out of one scrape after another.

I'm like a radio that is tuned into God's voice. If you become a Christian, you can tune into God's voice, too, and leave life's dilemmas up to Him. This is what I call real and true spirituality; total and utterly complete dependence on God.

Scripture backs this up in Proverbs 3:5-6. It says, "Trust in the LORD with all your heart and lean not on your own understanding; in all your ways acknowledge Him, and He will make your paths straight."

He makes my path straight through epiphanies. You may call it a "hunch," or a "still small voice," but I call it an "epiphany." This is a sudden striking or understanding of something, such as an important truth or decision. I've had many epiphanies in my lifetime that have been outstanding and memorable spiritual experiences. I believe all of these epiphanies have come from the Blessed Trinity, via the Holy Spirit. People often ask me if I think I have a direct pipeline to God, and my answer is always "Yes" and I add the comment that "If you are a Christian, you can also enjoy this same pipeline to God."

Jesus says in John 14:16, "I will ask the Father and He will give you another Counselor to be with you forever." This

Counselor, the Holy Spirit, gives me epiphanies. Perhaps the best Bible verse in favor of epiphanies is from Revelation 3:20, "Here I am! I stand at the door and knock. If anyone hears My voice and opens the door, I will come in and eat with him, and he with Me." Since inviting Christ to come in, I've continually sat and ate with Him, hearing His counsel through the Holy Spirit, receiving His epiphanies.

Here is a great example of an epiphany from God, a guiding voice that helped preserve my spiritual health. In 1995, my wife, Margaret Ann, and I were living in Fresno, California. I had been ministering in Sequoia National Forest and Sequoia/Kings Canyon National Parks since 1985, and I was a member of Belmont Christian Church in Fresno, a branch of the Independent Christian Church movement. Although the church, at that time, had been going through some internal struggles, Margaret Ann and I decided to keep attending. We retained our membership.

Yet, the conflict at Belmont Christian Church wasn't pretty. The pastor and associate pastor were having some doctrinal differences that finally led to the associate pastor resigning. Many church members smarted with hard feelings from the buffeting that occurred.

Within a year of the controversy, the pastor ended up resigning and accepted a pastorate in Oregon. Then, the church looked to *me* for leadership. I wasn't afraid to lead, but I felt the best thing to do initially was to encourage them to work things out amongst themselves. But in time, they *all* looked to me for leadership and I felt I simply could not let them down. This was a job that required me to operate at peak performance. I needed a strong spiritual foundation. So I reluctantly agreed to help with the future of the church, and fell to my knees, appealing to the God of the Bible to be my help and guide.

Shortly after, our congregation was approached by a sister congregation, the North Fresno Christian Church, to allow them to "merge" with us temporarily, while they were making plans to move north of Fresno and build new facilities to accommodate their growing membership. This Church was also an Independent Christian Church and was located just a few blocks from Belmont Christian Church.

The temporary merger was well-received by both congregations and all went well for three years. We all decided to change our name to Central Christian Church and slowly but surely, plans were made for new church facilities to be built on 20 acres of choice land north of Fresno. It was agreed that the new church would be called Northside Christian Church.

Those of us staying at Central Christian Church were faced with the difficult responsibility of finding new leadership. Again the Church looked to me for leadership, and again the challenge was formidable, to say the least. After some very difficult months of trials and errors, I suggested our church leaders meet with a very dear pastor friend, Rev. Bruce Mumper. Rev. Mumper was a Volunteer Pastor of Calvary Chapel in Fresno and made his living as a Physical Therapist. He was pastoring a church of some four hundred members, mostly young adults with lots of small children. They had no church facility of their own and were renting a school building on Sundays for their growing congregation.

It was "love at first sight" between our congregation and theirs, and soon we were worshipping and praising the Lord together on the campus of Central Christian Church. It was agreed to call the "new church" Calvary Chapel of Fresno, a Christian Church. It became obvious after a few weeks that the merging of the two congregations was a "marriage made in heaven." Everyone seemed to be thrilled and pleased with the move, especially Margaret Ann and I. Now comes the epiphany!

Margaret Ann and I were visiting in our living room with some devoted church members when I suddenly felt the Holy Spirit telling me it was time to move on. Move on? We had lived in our beautiful home in Fresno for twenty-one years and loved our home, our church, and our community and had made plans to live there until God called us to our eternal home!

As time went by and after much prayer and discussion, Margaret Ann and I decided this "epiphany" was truly a message from the Lord and now we need His direction on where to go from here.

After more prayer and discussion, we believed the Lord was leading us to move to Ojai, California, where our daughter, Pamela Petropulos, lived with her wonderful family. By way of confirmation from the Lord, within two hours after our Fresno home was listed on the Internet, a realtor called representing a young couple who had pre-qualified for a home loan and were ready to buy our particular house. Four hours later, our house was sold for what we were asking. Margaret Ann and I considered it a miracle and confirmation that we were in the center of God's perfect will.

Although I was spiritually drained from all of the events of the past few years in Fresno, I felt a confidence and satisfaction that I had listened to and obeyed God. I was confident the Lord did not want me to become involved with the new church situation in Fresno, but rather God was going to give me a new, spiritually refreshing life in Ojai. The move to Ojai was not without its own spiritual challenges, but I am more confident every day that this was a move prompted by the Lord. As a result, my obedience to that call has given me greater spiritual health today than if I had not listened to God, even, if for a moment, I faced a temporary physical health challenge.

The Physical Health Layer

Twelve years ago, in Ojai, I became very ill with some kind of virus. I experienced flu symptoms such as a fever, aches, chills and feeling sore all over. My medical doctor prescribed medicine, told me to go to bed, get plenty of sleep and rest, drink lots of liquids, and he ordered me to eat soft foods only throughout this illness. Despite following his orders, I felt terrible. I literally felt I was going to pass away.

After all the drama of the Fresno church struggles, our move to Ojai had not been easy. I'm sure the stress of that transition was a factor to my temporary ill health. Furthermore, I didn't have any opportunity to play golf or tennis or any organized sports for quite a while. My energy was down and there was not much I could do. Physically, I didn't feel very great, and I was just in my 70s.

But, here is where God kicked in and helped me out. I prayed a lot, and wanted to give up, but God wouldn't let me. He kept me in His care, even as I floundered. He told me

He would pull me through. I remembered James 5:14-15: "Is any one of you sick? He should call the elders of the church to pray over him and anoint him with oil in the name of the Lord. And the prayer offered in faith will make the sick person well; the Lord will raise him up. If he has sinned, he will be forgiven."

So, after I suffered for awhile, I asked my son-in-law Richard Petropulos, an elder of Ojai Valley Community Church, to come to our home and to pray for me and anoint me with oil in the name of the Lord. He was a fairly new Christian and a new elder. This was the first time he had ever done this, but he came with faith, fear, and trembling. He wasn't sure if God would move, but he complied with my request. As he prayed, I immediately felt some relief and had a calm assurance that in due time I would be well and once again enjoy great health. In about three days, I was out of bed and feeling great.

Not only did God hear Richard's prayers and improve my physical health, but our spiritual lives were also built up and strengthened. My physical need was an opportunity for God to move and improve my physical and spiritual health, as well as the spiritual health of my son-in-law. God, in His mercy, heard our prayers, and moved. These layers of health ideas were working. (Read more on the topic of "When Ill Health Strikes" in Chapter 13.)

According to **Figure 3** found in the preceding pages, the physical health layer lies directly on top of the spiritual health layer. The two are closely interconnected. If you are spiritually healthy, you are more likely to be physically healthy. Recent medical studies indicate that spiritual people exhibit fewer self-destructive behaviors (suicide, smoking, and drug and alcohol abuse, as examples), less stress, and a greater total life satisfaction.[2]

Don't be quick to dismiss the connection between spiritual health and physical health. You may ask, "What about all the obese Christians overeating at all their potlucks? What about the secular body builders or nutritionists? It seems they care more about their body than most Christians?" These are good questions, but they shouldn't be an excuse for neglecting the claims of Christ or for elevating your own physical health at the expense of your own soul. Body worship is idolatry and God won't stand for it, and ultimately, it won't serve you in the long run. Matthew 16:26 says, "What good will it be for a man if he gains the whole world, yet forfeits his soul? Or what can a man give in exchange for his soul?"

Muscles and appearance may get you somewhere in the world in the short term, but unless your health gains are a tool to be more effective in serving and worshiping God, then your quest for a better physical health layer is in vain. Proverbs 31:30 says, "Beauty is fleeting." Your physical health goals should be about making yourself a fit tool for God. And great physical health isn't about *perfect* health, as I can well attest. Even the fittest and healthiest among us face periodic illness and physical health struggles. But God is faithful and He can and will lead and guide you into greater physical health.

Mental Health Story

Just as my physical and spiritual health are interconnected, so too is my mental health with my spiritual and physical health. I can think truthfully and effectively (great mental health) when I have the mind of God (great spiritual health). I can think sharply and with efficiency (great mental health), when my body is functioning well (great physical health). After all, since being united with Christ in faith, I am an extension of Who and what God is. I live and move and have my being through God, and God gives substance to my body, to my life.

Without Them, I am like a piece of inanimate clay. At best, my mind would be the sum total of all my appetites. I'd be more like an animal running on instinct, seeking sheer survival. I'd be making decisions that benefit only me and not anyone else. And these decisions would lead quickly to my demise because I was not made for selfishness but community with God and with others. My selfishness would isolate me from God and others, and my mental capabilities would all be for naught.

Satan tries to persuade me I am okay without God, since God created me and gave me individuality, including a free will that enables me to be on my own, without any assistance from God. Yet, if I buy into Satan's ideas (as Eve did in the Garden of Eden and then persuaded Adam to do the same), I become mentally unhealthy, since it goes against the Plans of the Holy Trinity: God the Father, Son and Holy Spirit. God has a plan for how He wants human beings to think, act, talk, feel, etc. When humans rebel against God's plan and decisions, disastrous, unhealthy results occur: unhappiness, lack of peace, wrong decisions, misery, and death.

I can't pinpoint the exact day, but in 2003, I was standing in our kitchen and I felt a strong conviction and presence of the Holy Spirit. I was overwhelmed with the Holy Spirit trying to tell me I was falling short of being the man the

God of the Bible wanted me to be. Basically, I was refusing to accept my responsibility as the leader of my family, household and marriage. I was living and thinking a lie. My mental health was off because I was in error.

Humanly speaking, I was allowing my beloved wife to make final decisions in situations where we had major differences and/or where I was not 100% sure of my convictions. The Holy Spirit convicted me, right then and there, that He expected me to be the leader or decision-maker in every situation within our home and marriage. I was not to be a dictator or be insensitive to my wife's thoughts and feelings, but I was to make decisions based on what I honestly believed was God's Will as revealed to me via the Holy Spirit.

This was a major turning point in my life, in my marriage, and in my daily thoughts and actions. It also greatly affected my personal relationship with my beloved wife. Since that day, our marriage has been absolutely fantastic. I am much more at peace with myself and Margaret Ann has much more confidence in my family leadership. When we have a disagreement (which we have occasionally), I tell her I will think and pray about it before making any decisions, which she has learned to totally accept and respect.

We have decided this is according to the perfect plans of the God of the Bible and God is rewarding us daily with excellent health, and peace of mind, heart and soul. God assures me of the care He offers when I'm in the center of His will. If my spiritual health wasn't great, and my physical health wasn't great, I could have missed hearing out on the Holy Spirit that day in 2003. That prompting or conviction of God could have been the pizza talking instead, leading me in incorrect thinking and choices. I could have made wrong decisions, negatively affecting my health and the health of my marriage. I fully believe my mental health is better today because I now live every moment of every day in the wonderful will and plans of God the Father, Son, and Holy Spirit. Rebellion to God equals mental bondage. Obedience equals great mental health.

Emotional Health

I hope by now you are seeing how one layer of health affects another. By listening to the Holy Spirit and obeying His Word, I strengthen my spiritual and mental health and this in turn, affects my emotional health. As a minister and pastor, whose calling it seems, is to help assist churches for short seasons in life, my life has been uprooted on more than one occasion. I'm taken away from familiar surroundings and familiar people, many of whom I love. These moves could be a serious challenge to my emotional health. But, I learned long ago that no useful purpose is served by crying over circumstances I cannot control.

Our move from Fresno to Ojai, 200 miles South, brought many changes, some rather difficult. We left brothers and sisters in Christ, with whom we had established relationships over a period of many years. Some I had known, loved, and appreciated since childhood in the 1920s.

First and foremost was getting established in a good conservative, Bible-believing, Christ centered Church. Our Ojai family members were very active and involved in the Ojai Valley Community Church, so that question was easily answered.

Due to distance, we felt it best to sever our formal relationships with Central Christian Church (now Calvary Chapel), the Church of Sequoias (National Park Ministry), and the California Parks Ministry. We had no idea that our move to Ojai would signal the beginning of the end for the Church of the Sequoias. I had been involved with this ministry since the year 1929, when my father helped start it.

The Ranger Naturalists in Sequoia and Kings Canyon National Parks were quick to take advantage of our move to Ojai by ordering our Church of Sequoias Parsonage (a 30 by 12 foot mobile home) out of Giant Forest in Sequoia National Park, and taking over all of our Guest Minister Cabins, which we had built and paid for with Church of Sequoias donations. Without these "homes" there was no way the Church of Sequoias could continue, and the ministry in the two parks was soon turned over to a national organization called, Christian Ministry in the National Parks.

This was heart-breaking, especially for me, and required some major adjustments mentally, spiritually, emotionally, and physically. Some measure of guilt was experienced, as well as resentment toward the Ranger Naturalists, who were not usually supportive of our Church of Sequoias Christian Ministry. Most felt that the National Parks were designed and existed for the sole purpose of protecting and appreciating some of our nation's natural resources (trees, flowers, plants, rivers, streams, lakes, geysers, wild-life, etc.) and viewed religious activities as an intrusion and even violation of the goals of the Department of Interior. Therefore it became a real challenge for me to put all of this behind me and press on ahead.

The words of the Apostle Paul in Philippians 3:12-16 were very helpful to me. "I press on to take hold of that for which Christ Jesus took hold of me. Brothers, I do not consider myself yet to have taken hold of it. But one thing I do: forgetting what is behind and straining toward what is ahead, I press on toward the goal to win the prize for which God has called me heavenward in Christ Jesus. All of us who are mature should take such a view of things. And if on some point you think differently, that too God will make clear to you. Only let us live up to what we have already attained." I believed I had been obedient to my responsibility for the Ministry, and my responsibility ended when I moved to Ojai.

A big part of emotional health is keeping your expectations in check. Emotionally unwell people expect their lives to be different, and when they don't get what they want, they pout, wail, complain and get depressed. As long as you call this world your home, life will not be fair and it will not give you what you want.

God isn't a vending machine in that He gives you what you want. He gives you what you need. And, mercifully, He can also give you contentment, even in the middle of the darkest hours. Sometimes God changes your expectations.

Sometimes He tells us to wait. Other times, He tells us to double our efforts and determination. Always, we should be praying like Jesus when He faced crucifixion, "not My will, but Yours be done" (Luke 22:42).

And when all the praying is done and you have been obedient to God as much as you understand, you look at what has happened and you praise God. You praise Him because

God asks us to "*give thanks* in all circumstances, for this is God's will for you in Christ Jesus" (1 Thess. 5:18). You praise Him when you got the raise and when you didn't. You also praise Him when you find out you'll be stuck in your boring job for awhile and you praise Him when you get a new and better job. In good and bad, God is to be praised.

Good Health is a Choice

Though the God of the Bible sustains me, leads me and guides me, my great health is still a choice. God has given me free will and I can choose to follow Him (leading to great health) or disobey Him (leading to poor health). Proverbs 13:4 says, "The sluggard craves and gets nothing, but the desires of the diligent are fully satisfied." I don't want to stand before God one day and say I made excuses on my health. Even Ben Franklin once observed, "The person who is good at excuse-making is seldom good at anything else." I want God to say to me, "Well done, good and faithful servant" (Matt. 25:23).

Blaming others for your poor health isn't going to help you become any healthier either. President Calvin Coolidge said, "Don't expect to build up the weak by pulling down the strong." Only you can strengthen your overall health by taking responsibility for it. Those who are already healthy and strong should not be envied or scorned, but praised and esteemed. They are your role models and can help inspire you and give you advice on how to achieve great health.

A person of personal responsibility owns up to his or her own failures in poor health. If you aren't eating right, admit it. If you aren't exercising well, don't make excuses for being a couch-potato. And if you have been ignoring God or contenting yourself with spiritual lies, tell yourself and others, "I don't know much, I'd like to learn." The power to great health is in your hands, but only God the Father, Son and Holy Spirit can safely lead you and guide you throughout your life's journey.

In the next section, ***Layer One: Spiritual Health***, I'll begin to explore in greater detail the ins and outs of improving your spiritual health. Great health and a great life begin with a great relationship with the Father God of the Bible, His Precious Son and His Blessed Holy Spirit.

Footnotes

1. http://charactercounts.org/sixpillars.html.
2. http://kidshealth.org/parent/emotions/feelings/spirituality.html.

Layer One: Spiritual Health

Chapter 3
Living In God's Truth

Teach me Your way, O LORD, and I will walk in Your truth; give me an undivided heart, that I may fear Your name.
- Psalm 86:11

Jesus answered, I am the way and the truth and the life. No one comes to the Father except through Me. - John 14:6

Every builder knows that a firm foundation is essential for keeping structures upright, safe and secure. A foolish builder might use flimsy, shifty materials, or cut corners on what's right in order to save money and increase his profit. However, there are no shortcuts or savings when foundations crumble, compromising the integrity of the building. The work will have to be done right, incurring further time and expense.

A firm spiritual foundation is no different. If I had built my spiritual foundation on anything else but the solid rock of the God of the Bible, I would have been swept away at the slightest bit of adversity. Thankfully, I learned to build my spiritual foundation on the Truth of God relatively early in my life.

It was in July, 1946. I had been singing with the Country Church of Hollywood Quartet (Goose Creek Quartet, as heard on the radio) and the Old Fashioned Revival Hour Quartet. (These were the same quartets. They just had different names.) After a successful run of singing at various venues, I felt very sure of myself. I felt like I had secured God's favor with my excellent works. I felt I had become a superior human being through my own righteousness. Then the top tenor, Bill MacDougall, confronted me with the error of my thinking.

After a radio broadcast, he showed me the truth of Isaiah 64:6, "All of us have become like one who is unclean, and all our righteous acts are like filthy rags; we all shrivel up like a leaf and like the wind our sins sweep us away." That verse tore at the core of my being. He had taken a hammer to the foundation of good works that I had built within me, and it turned my world upside down.

Up to that point, through my 24 years of living, I based my spiritual foundations on *all* the great decisions and behaviors *I* had made. I always thought the God of the Bible appreciated the fact that I had given my life to Jesus Christ at age 9. I boasted that He must be proud of the fact that I had tried to live the Christian life to the best of my ability. I had denied myself things like sex, tobacco, alcohol, profanity, harmful foods or beverages, etc. for the sake of my precious Savior. Furthermore, I could say I regularly attended church (even while in the Seabees during WW II). I defended Jesus Christ and His Church when anyone spoke against the God of the Bible, and I practiced high ethical standards. In other words, I thought of myself as the perfect Christian. I had built my spiritual foundation on self-acclaim, pride, and self-centeredness. I had virtually lost all my appreciation and dependence on what Jesus Christ had done for me on the Cross of Calvary.

My first reaction to Bill and the Word he brought to me was anger and disbelief. But in the days that followed, I had a chance to think and reflect on what he had told me. I realized he spoke from the Bible, the inerrant Word of Truth. He wasn't speaking his opinion, or his own thoughts. Rather, he had spoken to me the Word of God, and it cut me to the quick. With those piercing words, Bill began to rebuild my foundation with Truth. I slowly began to realize that I needed a new foundation. I needed to understand what it truly meant to accept Jesus Christ as Lord and Savior. I needed Christ to be the foundation of my life, not my own good works.

Soon thereafter, God revealed His Atoning, Redeeming work for me by reminding me of the lyrics of such old hymns as "In the Cross of Christ I Glory," "When I Survey the Wondrous Cross," "The Old Rugged Cross," "Down at the Cross Where My Savior Died," and "At the Cross, At the Cross Where I First Saw the Light," etc. These lyrics reminded me of the enormous price Christ paid to establish my holiness. I realized that anything I had done for God was cheap in comparison to Christ's sacrificial work for me.

I saw the great truths in scriptures with fresh eyes. The Apostle Paul said in 1 Corinthians 2:2, "For I resolved to know nothing while I was with you except Jesus Christ and Him crucified." Scriptures on the Atonement and Christ's death on the cross leapt out from the page and convicted me of my error. So, from that point forward, my life became more Christ-centered instead of Dick Brown centered. I relied more on God's Holy and Written Word (the Bible) instead of my own thoughts, feelings and education and conclusions. To this day, I praise and thank the God of the Bible for speaking to me through His servant, Bill MacDougall, on that summer morning in July of 1946.

My life, all these years later, is radically different because my foundation was rebuilt on truth instead of lies. In fact, a firm and Biblically correct spiritual foundation is essential to great spiritual health. As evidenced from the story above, I believe a correct spiritual foundation starts with genuine faith.

The Importance of Faith

Faith is elemental. Hebrews 11:6 says, "Without faith it is impossible to please God, because anyone who comes to Him must believe that He exists and that He rewards those who earnestly seek Him." Woe to the unfaithful, those who displease God. When faith in God is discarded, for the Christian and non-Christian alike, hope for great health in this life or in the hereafter evaporates!

The best definition of Christian faith I've ever run across can be found in Proverbs 3:5-6: "Trust in the Lord with all your heart and lean not on your own understanding; in all your ways acknowledge Him and He will make your paths straight." God has shown His straight paths for me since 1946. I daily surrender my mind, heart, soul and body to God the Father, God the Son (Jesus), and God the Holy Spirit, otherwise known as the God of The Bible.

Surrendering your heart and will to God may seem difficult because it involves trust in an unseen entity, but the practice of daily surrender and faith in God yields great dividends of great health. When you live a life of faith, you give control of your life over to a higher power. You give up all your rights, but in the process, you gain God's protection, guidance and fellowship with Him. Additionally, you surrender your right to worry. (Jesus says in Matthew 6:31, "So do not worry, saying, 'What shall we eat?' or 'What shall we drink?' or 'What shall we wear?' For the pagans run after all these things, and your heavenly Father knows that you need them.") The God of the Bible is a God that promises to meet all your needs if you trust solely in Him. Through surrender, you also have access to an all-powerful God that hears your prayers. (Jesus tells us in Mark 11:24: "Therefore I tell you, whatever you ask for in prayer, believe that you have received it, and it will be yours.") God, furthermore, opens up to you a whole legacy of wisdom, truth, and statutes for life. The Bible and all the records of God blessing His saints throughout history are available to us. We can also learn from and be inspired by the saints alive today, who give encouraging testimony to His greatness and His steadfast care.

We also have a forgiving, understanding God, who listens when we have doubts. He listens when our faith slips. We know this because in Mark 9:20-26, Jesus tells a father, whose son suffers from demonic convulsions, "Everything is possible for him who believes. Immediately the boy's father exclaimed, 'I do believe; help me overcome my unbelief!'" The father didn't have belief, but he wanted it. Jesus responded with favor on the man and cast the demons out. Jesus cared about the health of this man's family, merely because the man said he wanted a faith he lacked. Wow! That's some God – this Jesus Christ.

Faith in Jesus

If faith in God is the foundation to good health, then Jesus Christ is the mortar to that foundation. He's the object of that faith. When I accepted Him as my personal Lord and Savior in March of 1931, He gave me many great promises, promises that are available to all who put their faith and trust in Him. Jesus promises to take care of my total health. Jesus promises to take care of my physical health when He says He will never leave me hungry or thirsty (John 6:35). He also promises to heal me (Matt. 9:22). He takes care of our mental health as our instructor (Matt. 21:6) and teacher (Matt. 19:16). He's the caretaker of our emotional health as our comforter (Matt. 5:4) and peace (John 20:26). He is the ultimate health-giver when He promises eternal life (John 6:51). In short, Jesus promises great health to all who put their trust in Him, both in this life and in the life to come.

Some may question Jesus as a health giver when chronic illnesses linger. People ask, "Where is God when my family member is dying of cancer, or suffering from some other terrible debilitating disease?" I'll go into great detail answering these questions in "Chapter 15: When Ill Health Strikes," but there are special times and circumstances where God withholds His healing power for a time in order to display a greater work. In other words, your suffering may be achieving a higher purpose. Job followed God and he was not spared from calamity. Even God's son, Jesus, suffered life-long persecution and then death on the cross. God's ways are not our ways, and your lack of health may be an instrument for a greater work of God. (If you don't believe me, ask people like Joni Erickson Tada, a paraplegic who has a worldwide ministry to the disabled. God is faithful and has kept His promises to her.)

Yes. God keeps His promises! His promise recorded in Matthew 6:33-34 has been, without a doubt, the overall guiding principle of my life and I refer to it daily to remind me of why God created me and the basic purpose of my existence: "But seek first His kingdom and His righteousness, and all these things will be given to you as well. Therefore, do not worry about tomorrow for tomorrow will worry about itself. Each day has enough trouble of its own."

Faith in Christ is not necessarily an easy insurance plan for great health. If it was, everyone would gladly pay the premium. Jesus said, "If anyone would come after Me, he must deny himself and take up his cross daily and follow Me" (Luke 9:23). The cost of Jesus' health care plan is nothing less than denying yourself and surrendering to Him completely. Jesus was and is a challenge to those who would dare listen to believe.

In fact, before indiscriminately believing in Him, consider some of the claims Jesus made that caused many of His contemporaries to insist He was insane, a blasphemer and in league with Satan himself! Some of these claims included:

- "I am the Way, the Truth and the Life. No one comes to the Father except by Me." (John 14:6)

- "The Father and I are One." (John 10:30)

- "I tell you the truth, unless you eat the flesh of the Son of Man and drink His blood, you have *no life* in you. Whoever eats My flesh and drinks My blood has eternal life, and I will raise him up at the last day. For My flesh is real food and My blood is real drink. Whoever eats My flesh and drinks My blood remains in Me, and I in him." (John 6:53-56)

- "Therefore I tell you, whatever you ask for *in prayer*, believe that you have received it, and it will be yours." (Mark 11:24)

Throughout my life, I studied these claims very seriously. I've concluded that despite how crazy or outlandish these claims are, they are altogether true. If you are just coming to Christ or if you are having a hard time understanding some of these claims, it's important to remember 2 Corinthians 3:6 which says, "the letter kills but the Spirit gives *life*." If you get bogged down and sidetracked by some of Jesus' more difficult teachings, you may be tempted to not believe. Always ask God to send you the Holy Spirit to help you understand what He is trying to say to you. He can help you fully understand the meaning and application of any scripture verse or verses. Taking certain scriptures literally instead of spiritually can "kill" the great spiritual truth God is trying to convey to you. God's Word is there to give you life, not confuse you, but to challenge and encourage you. The Holy Spirit can help you understand and appreciate more of what Jesus is saying through His Word. The adventure of faith is often a straight path and a green pasture, but it can also be a rough sea and a dark valley. Thank God for Jesus, to be there for us to constantly be our companion and guide no matter what terrain we are on.

The Truth of God's Love

One of the most popular Bible verses ever written about Jesus is John 3:16. "For God so loved the world that He gave His one and only Son, that whoever believes in Him shall not perish but have eternal life." This is the Good News of the Gospel and it is a Scripture to embrace and love for all time. However, the verse has been abused and mistreated throughout the years. People say, "Yeah. I believe in Jesus," and they think that in itself is a free pass to heaven. They reason, "If I just give mental assent to the existence of Jesus, I can do as I please. I can sin freely. I can choose to not follow Jesus and He'll let me into heaven. After all, God is love (1 John 2:5) right? He has to forgive me, right?" Wrong! God is love but His love is *not* unconditional.

I firmly believe that health cannot exist without Truth. The two are inseparable. The more Truth we have in our minds, bodies, hearts, and souls, the better chance we have of being healthy spiritually, physically, mentally and emotionally. I am really not comfortable with using the phrase "God's Unconditional Love." Many scriptures in both the Old and New Testaments imply or state directly that there are circumstances and situations where God does not practice love but rather hatred, anger and destruction. His Wrath is manifested in ways that defy a loving attitude toward those who are on the receiving end. Let's take a look at some of these scriptures:

- **Exodus 4:14** - "Then the LORD's *anger* burned against Moses." (Here, God is angry with one of the most beloved religious figures of all time, Moses.)

- **Exodus 32:9** - "Now leave Me alone so that my *anger* may burn against them and that I may *destroy* them." (Here, God wants to wipe out His chosen people, the Israelites.)

- **Deuteronomy 6:15 - "**For the LORD your God, who is among you, is a jealous God and His anger will burn against you, and He will *destroy* you from the face of the land." (This is a not-so-pleasant fact that God wished to remind His people.)

- **Micah 5:10** - "In that day," declares the LORD, "I will *destroy* your horses from among you and demolish your chariots." (God's hatred includes ruining even animals and property.)

- **Matthew 10:28 - "**Do not be afraid of those who kill the body but cannot kill the soul. Rather, be afraid of the One who can *destroy* both soul and body in hell." (Jesus gets into the destruction business.)

- **James 4:12 - "**There is only One Lawgiver and Judge, the One who is able to save and destroy." (The apostle James gets in to speaking some hard truth. The One he speaks of is God.)

These verses are mainly directed at believers, those who have faith in the God of the Bible. If so much destruction is available to the believer, imagine what God might have in store for the rebellious, defiant, and the unrepentant!

I've become convinced that God has a dual nature (love and hate) and this dual nature is often manifested in the human beings He has created. When the Bible says God hated Esau (Mal. 1:3), we can assume He also loved him in that He provided him with the basic necessities of life (food, clothing, shelter, air, etc.). But how do you explain away the written word that God hated Esau? You can't! Hence, God was both loving and hating at the same time.

Most people do not like to hear of the other side of God's nature and character because they prefer to only hear of the positive side, such as love and forgiveness and mercy. I can't remember ever hearing a sermon on God's Wrath, except those I would occasionally preach. Invariably, when I would preach on God's Wrath and Judgment and Eternal Hell, there would be many objections and comments such as: "I don't come to church to hear messages like this. They are so very negative. I come to church to hear good and positive things about God and life on this earth."

Jonathan Edwards, the well-known preacher/evangelist of the 1700s, is perhaps best remembered for his famous sermon: "Sinners in the Hands of an Angry God." It has been reported that some people listening to this sermon would literally hold onto their seats for fear of being cast into Hell at that moment. Edwards ends the sermon with one final appeal, "Therefore let everyone that is out of Christ, now awake and fly from the wrath to come." Without explicitly saying, Edwards indirectly gives a sense of hope to those currently out of Christ. Only by returning to Christ can one escape the stark fate outlined by Edwards. I don't know what would happen if this sermon were to be preached in the church of today. I doubt that it would be well-received because most of us seem to be caught up with this idea of God's Unconditional Love.

The Bible makes it clear that God is the same yesterday, today, and forever. Therefore, the God of the Old Testament is the same as the God of the New Testament. Man has always been and forever shall be saved by the grace of God, not by personal works lest any man should boast. In Old Testament times, man was required to make certain animal and bird sacrifices in order to fulfill all the requirements of God's Laws, but God always made it clear that making these sacrifices alone did not fulfill all the requirements. God required true repentance, not just outward, but inward as well, before He would accept the sacrifices. This is confirmed through the Bible verse, Psalm 51:17, "The sacrifices of God are a broken spirit; a broken and contrite heart, O God, You will not despise." God doesn't want you to merely go through the motions. He wants your heart in the right place. So, with regard to sacrifice, we see a form of conditional love on the part of God. Put in another way, we see conditions that had to be met before God's Love would be manifested. In this case, it's humility.

Obedience

God also requires obedience if we are to *fully* experience His love. 1 John 2:5 says, "But if anyone obeys His Word, God's love is truly made complete in Him." God won't reveal His full love, unless obedience is practiced.

Furthermore, Jesus states in John 14:23: "If anyone loves

Me, he will obey My teaching. My Father will love him and We will come to him and make Our home with him." It seems clear to me that God puts a condition on this promise of love by using the word "If." We must obey God to receive His love. We also read in Matthew 13:53-58 of Jesus *not* doing many miracles in His home-town due to the lack of faith on the part of the townspeople. No doubt He loved his townspeople, but His expression of that Love was certainly limited and conditional in Nazareth.

I know when I obey God and thank Him for His Grace, I sense His love more strongly than when I am proud and following my own counsel. Obedience to God is essential for the great health I enjoy. My dad used to say to me, "I'd rather you obey me than love me." My mother was shocked at this statement, but it was very important to him that I learned obedience because it was so important. Obedience to my earthly father led to obedience to my Heavenly Father.

My dad loved me, no question about that (though at times I doubted it due to his emphasis on obedience). He deeply cared about my thoughts and feelings toward him but he cared more about the God of the Bible. He refused to be distracted by anything that might interfere with his assignment from his Creator, even if it was his own family. God was his #1 priority, and he wanted me and everyone in my family to know that.

I did not dare disobey my dad as long as he was on this earth (I was age 12 when he passed away) and it was only after he passed away that I began to have warm and good feelings toward him, which have increased daily since December of 1934. My main point is that God has created us for Himself and for His Pleasure and for His use in carrying on His Work. With Him we are something and without Him we are nothing. I am, in a way, an extension of God, created in His Image, like Him in many ways, only falling far short of actually being Him. Human relationships mean a lot to me but are dwarfed in comparison to my relationship with my Creator and His Son and His Holy Spirit. And the better my relationship is with the God of the Bible, the better my relationship with other people are in general, and certain ones in particular.

Obeying God yields dividends on this earth and in the life to come. What health benefit is it to obey God? Spiritually speaking, I've discovered that no one ever dies but we all go on living somewhere else. Also, I've been learning how to conquer fear, guilt, hate, feelings of inferiority, depression, over- and under-confidence, and I'm realizing the extreme importance of recognizing others. I'm exercising the gifts of the Holy Spirit (gifts God has given me), taking God at His Word in the Holy Scriptures, and I'm listening to the Holy Spirit's leading. I'm realizing the purpose of evil on this earth and why God has and continues to allow it. I'm realizing that I can do all things through Christ Who strengthens me, realizing that in all things God is working for my good because I love Him and have accepted His calling. I'm learning to recognize Satan and I'm learning from God how to defeat the ruler of this world and the father of all lies. I'm learning *not* to follow *my* heart since my heart outside of Christ is deceitful and wicked above all things, but I'm learning to follow the *new* heart and mind that has been given to me since I've accepted Jesus as Lord and Savior.

Make sure your spiritual foundation is safe and secure. Obey God and stand on His truth. This will give you great health, and secure your spiritual foundation when adversity strikes. With such a strong foundation, your other health layers: physical, mental and emotional, stand the best chance to also become secure and strong.

Believing in God's Truth is the best way to secure that firm spiritual foundation. One way to help you embrace God's Truth is to discern Satan's lies. Oh yes. The Devil is as alive and real today as he was during Biblical times. He and his demons are out there, ready to steal, kill, and destroy all those who would wittingly or unwittingly succumb to his lures. Discerning and rejecting Satan's lies are just as important as standing on God's Truth in securing a strong spiritual foundation. They are so important that I've dedicated a whole chapter on it. Let's learn about your spiritual enemy and what we can do to combat his evil plans against you, preventing you from enjoying excellent health.

Chapter 4
Denying Satan's Lies

He replied, I saw Satan fall like lightning from heaven. - Luke 10:18

The great dragon was hurled down—that ancient serpent called the devil, or Satan, who leads the whole world astray. He was hurled to the earth, and his angels with him.
- Revelations 12:9

There are three different beliefs about Satan that people hold today. Some people simply refuse to believe in Satan and are therefore in his grip. Others *do* believe in Satan but have wittingly or unwittingly succumbed to some or many of his lies. And finally, there are others who believe that Satan is real, is dangerous, and are up to his tricks. They have consciously chosen to reject Satan and instead, have chosen to remain in the grip and grace of God. Which type of person are you?

As a believer in the God of the Bible, I am one who believes Satan does exist. I know he is altogether evil and he seems to be working overtime these days to spread his lies. The Bible calls Satan the Father of lies. One day, Jesus was talking to some Jews, who had once believed in Him, and He told them, “You belong to your father, the devil, and you want to carry out your father’s desire. He was a murderer from the beginning, not holding to the truth, for there is no truth in him. When he speaks, he speaks his native language, for he is a liar and the fathcr of lies” (John 8:44). Notice that Jesus exposes one of Satan’s greatest lies, namely, that all human beings who live (or have lived) on this earth are “children of God.” The truth is that some people “belong to their father, the devil, and want to carry out their father’s desires.”

To recognize God and His truth, you must be aware that there is an enemy: Satan, his helpers and their lies. Many people do not believe in God, let alone Satan, but let me assure you, both are very real. In John 10:10 it says, “Who is this adversary, this Father of lies, the enemy who comes to steal, kill and destroy?”

The Apostle John writes in Revelation 12:7-9 “And there was war in heaven. Michael and his angels fought against the dragon (Satan) and the dragon and his angels fought back. But he was not strong enough and they lost their place in heaven. The great dragon was hurled down - that ancient serpent, called the devil or Satan, who leads the whole world astray. He was hurled to the earth and his angels (demons) with him.” Satan was, we assume, originally created by God to worship God and do God’s bidding. But, like us humans, angels were given free-will and Satan exercised his free-will to rebel against God. The God of the Bible, being Holy, had no choice but to banish Satan and his angels from Heaven.

Even a casual reader of the Bible cannot question the existence of Satan, provided the reader believes the Bible is the Word of God. If a reader picks up a Bible and chooses to believe portions of it and disbelieve others, what standard is there for judging any theological point? These readers give themselves a loophole for doubt by saying the Bible "contains" the Word of God, rather than "is" the Word of God. I'm convinced that *my* good health is directly related to the fact that I believe the Bible *is* the Word of God. When I read it, I am reading what *God* has written through a number of chosen men, beginning with Moses in the Book of Genesis and ending with the Apostle John in the Book of Revelation. If I reject some of it, I must reject all of it. It is an all or nothing deal, as far as I'm concerned.

So, in regards to Satan, the Bible implies though does not explicitly say so, that he was created by God, and fell from Heaven. I must believe that. And, since the Bible says he is the father of lies, then that is also something I must stand behind. Satan, I'm convinced, is behind *all* evil just like God is behind *all* good. Nevertheless, all mankind is created in the image of God and is given the right to make choices. It is very easy and very convenient for people to blame Satan for any and all wrongs they commit. But, by doing this, people avoid accepting responsibility for their own thoughts, words, and deeds.

The God of the Bible tells us we must believe that He "is" in order to really believe, trust, and obey Him. This is the essence of faith. In a sort of reverse way, the same is also true about Satan. In order to reject Satan and his lies, we must believe that he "is" and then we must believe what the Bible says about him. Outside sources may say it is okay to follow Satan, that he is good and will help you get what you want and need. Nonsense! Only the record of Holy Scripture accurately and dependably accounts Satan's history and character. It is pointless and non-productive to try and learn about who he is from non-authoritative texts.

The Apostle Paul writes in 2 Corinthians 11:13-15, "For such men are false apostles, deceitful workmen, masquerading as apostles of Christ. And no wonder, for Satan himself masquerades as an angel of light. It is not surprising, then, if his servants masquerade as servants of righteousness. Their end will be what their actions deserve."

It is important to recognize Satan and his lies so that you will not be ensnared by them. Believing them will be detrimental to your temporal and eternal health! Satan's lies are legion and I can't possibly deal with all of them in this book, but what I can do is highlight some of his most obvious lies that the Holy Spirit has allowed me to understand and to overcome. Let's look at and examine some of the most common lies that Satan propagates today.

Common Lies Believed Today

Lie #1: Satan does not exist. Neither does Hell.

Satan loves to convince people he doesn't exist. If he is successful with that lie, he can do his evil work "undercover," without detection or blame. He is a master at counterfeit and disguise and masquerading. In the New International Version of the Bible, the name Satan is mentioned 47 times. The devil is mentioned an additional 35 times, and demon (or demons) is stated 80 times. All of these occurrences are given in reference to actual, created beings that have influence over mankind.

The awful truth about Hell, found in Revelation 20:15, says, "If anyone's name was not found written in the book of life, he was thrown into the lake of fire." The lake of fire is Hell – a place void of the presence and grace of God. To find out how you can have your name written in the book of life, look at the appendix to read the section "How You can Enjoy Great Eternal Health."

I recently had a discussion with a golfing buddy, who is

a professing Christian, but does not believe in Satan or Hell. He claims everybody will eventually end up in heaven with our Wonderful Creator and all His Family. If you quote the Bible at him, he'll shake his head because this man rejects the Truth of Scripture. He believes the Bible is the word of man, and not the Word of God. The best I can do is pray the Holy Spirit will lead him to repentance, but for now, this man has accepted a lie.

1 Peter 5:8 says, "Be self-controlled and alert. Your enemy the devil prowls around like a roaring lion looking for someone to devour." My friend above has already been attacked and consumed by the enemy. If you know Satan exists, you can watch for him and you can remain on guard to protect yourself when he does strike.

Lie #2: You can enter Heaven if you are a good person or We are all going to Heaven.

So many people today believe that there are multiple roads to heaven. They think that all religions are ultimately the same. They think if you are a good _____________ (fill in the blank with any religion) that God will accept you into heaven, or if you don't believe in heaven, that you'll receive good karma or be reincarnated to the next best being or achieve some kind of eternal reward anyway.

The Bible says differently. Jesus said, "I am the way and the truth and the life. No one comes to the Father except through Me" (John 14:6). He also said in Mark 16:16, "Whoever believes and is baptized will be saved." Just to make it clear so that there is no room for doubt, Jesus adds in the same verse, "but whoever does not believe will be condemned." It doesn't look like there is any wiggle room here. Faith in Christ is essential for salvation.

Besides, if you could get to heaven by your good works and by being a good ____________ (fill in the blank with any religion), then the death and resurrection of Christ was for nothing. Christ needed to be God and He needed to die and rise again to break the curse of death that Satan brought to this earth upon Adam and Eve when they first sinned in the Garden of Eden. God's redemptive grace is not cheap. It's costly. Nothing less than the spilled blood of Christ is sufficient to pay the entry price for our ticket into heaven. Those who reject this ticket and how it was paid for will not enter the Kingdom of Heaven. Jesus said, "Enter through the narrow gate. For wide is the gate and broad is the road that leads to destruction, and many enter through it. But small is the gate and narrow the road that leads to life and only a few find it" (Matt. 7:13-15).

Lie #3: The Bible really isn't the Word of God, and is therefore, not authoritative Truth.

In order to believe in Christ and His atoning work, and also the existence of the devil and his work of destruction, you first must believe that the Bible is the authoritative Word of God and Truth. If Satan can convince you that the Bible isn't really the authoritative Word of God, then any theological or moral Truth it dictates is really up for grabs. It's religion *a la carte* – pick and choose off the menu what you like and don't accept the rest.

I accept all 66 books of the Bible (Genesis through Revelation). I accept the historical fact that these 66 books became our official Bible after much discussion and prayer on the part of many Christian leaders. These leaders were selected by Roman Emperor Constantine and ordered to meet together at what came to be known as the First Council of Nicaea in 325 AD. From this event came the Nicene Creed, a statement of faith which is still declared and believed in by Christians today. (See appendix for a copy of the Nicene Creed in modern language.)

The primary reason Emperor Constantine ordered the Council to meet was to settle the questionable Arian views of the Trinity, but he also wanted to determine once and for all which books were to be included in what would soon be called the Holy Bible. If any book was insufficient in its historicity and content, it was not included in the Holy Bible, and therefore could not be proclaimed as God's Holy Word.

I believe God was with those early Christian leaders and this Council of Nicaea, and that God's Holy Spirit guided them in the decisions they made. It is really quite mind-boggling to believe that these 66 books contain the words of Almighty God Himself, and I applaud everyone who has taken a step of faith to believe these books are the authoritative Word of the God. For me, it was a decision I made gradually from the day I was born until the day I accepted Christ. But being convinced of their power and might, I now more than ever believe in the authority of the Bible.

Hebrews 4:12-13 says, "For the Word of God is living and active, sharper than any double-edged sword, it penetrates even to dividing soul and spirit, joints and marrow; it judges the thoughts and attitudes of the heart. Nothing in all creation is hidden from God's sight. Everything is uncovered and laid bare before the eyes of Him to whom we must give account." A double-edge sword is designed for maximum cutting ability. It is used often for fighting and beheading. It is lethal and will kill those who would fight against its power.

I believe the Bible answers all the questions we need in order to live a successful life that God has given us. I believe this because the Bible is the Word of God. But if one does not believe that, any truth, any code of life, any standard of living is equally valid.

All theological discussion must stem from the authority of the Bible. The questions must be asked: Is the Bible authoritative? Is it the Word of God or the Word of man? The answer to these questions will determine your temporal and eternal health.

Other Lies Believed Today

Many other lies of Satan are believed today, but I believe they all fall under the categories of one of the three major lies listed above. If neither Satan, nor Hell, nor any particular way to Heaven, nor Absolute Truth exists, then anything can be believed. Below are several other popular lies believed today by the masses. (They are by no means all of Satan's lies but they can be found on the lips of many today.) Since I believe the Bible is the authoritative Word of God, I've also included some Bible verses as a Truthful response to these lies. These verses are not the total argument against these lies, but they are a starting point to show you that the Bible does have an answer to counter all these lies.

- The real goal of life is happiness and anything and everything that makes a person happy must be okay! (**Prov. 14:12** - "There is a way that seems right to a man, but in the end it leads to death.")

- It is not necessary to be born again. (**John 3:7** - "Jesus said, 'You should not be surprised at My saying, You must be born again.'")

- Life on this earth is all there is. (**Dan. 12:2** - "Multitudes who sleep in the dust of the earth will awake: some to everlasting life, others to shame and everlasting contempt." **Heb. 9:27-28** - "Just as man is destined to die once, and after that to face judgment, so Christ was sacrificed once to take away the sins of many people; and He will appear a second time, not to bear sin but to bring salvation to those who are waiting for Him.")

- I need to be selfish and get all I can out of life while I'm here. (**Matt. 6:25** -"For whoever wants to save his life will lose it, but whoever loses his life for Me will find it.")

- What I've done really isn't that bad. I'm not a sinner. (**Rom. 3:23** - "All have sinned and have fallen short of the Glory of God.")

- Same-sex marriage is okay if two people love each other! (**Gen. 2:24** - "For this reason a man will leave his father and mother and be united to his wife, and they will become one flesh," and **Lev. 18:22** - "Do not lie with a man as one lies with a woman; that is detestable.")

- Abortion is okay if the mother-to-be decides for any reason whatsoever that she does not want her baby. (**Ps. 139: 13-14** - "For you created my inmost being; You knit me together in my mother's womb. I praise

You because I am fearfully and wonderfully made.")

- After I die, I'll be reincarnated into something else. (**Heb. 9:27** - "Man is destined to die once, and after that to face judgment." **Matt. 25:41** - "Then He will say to those on His left, 'Depart from me, you who are cursed, into the eternal fire prepared for the devil and his angels.'")

- Man can't possibly know God since the gap between God and man is too great! (**John 15:15** - "I no longer call you servants, because a servant does not know his master's business. Instead, I have called you friends, for everything that I learned from my Father I have made known to you." **John 14:23** - "Jesus replied, 'If anyone loves Me, he will obey My teaching. My Father will love him, and We will come to him and make Our home with him.'")

- Marriage is a democracy. The idea of the man being the head of his household is chauvinistic and that order belongs back in the Dark Ages and not in this Age of Enlightenment. (**Eph. 5:22-25** - "Wives, submit to your husbands as to the Lord. For the husband is the head of the wife as Christ is the head of the church, His body, of which He is the Savior. Now as the church submits to Christ, so also wives should submit to their husbands in everything. Husbands, love your wives, just as Christ loved the church and gave Himself up for her.")

- It is very wrong to discipline children as it might prevent them from being free to be themselves and from freely expressing themselves and from being the persons God has created them to be. (**Prov. 13:24** - "He who spares the rod hates his son, but he who loves him is careful to discipline him." **Heb. 12:6** - "The Lord disciplines those He loves, and He punishes everyone He accepts as a son." **Prov. 3:11-12** - "My son, do not despise the LORD's discipline and do not resent His rebuke, because the LORD disciplines those He loves, as a father the son He delights in.")

- Becoming a Christian and living the Christian life takes most or all of the fun out of life. (**Job 8:21** - "He will yet fill your mouth with laughter and your lips with shouts of joy." **John 10:10** - "The thief comes only to steal and kill and destroy; I have come that they may have life, and have it to the full." **Prov. 17:22** - "A cheerful heart is good medicine, but a crushed spirit dries up the bones.")

- Follow your heart and you can't go wrong. (**Jer. 17: 9** - "The heart is deceitful above all things and beyond cure. Who can understand it?")

- Your parent's thoughts are old-fashioned and outdated. (**Prov. 4:1** - "Listen, my sons, to a Father's instruction; pay attention and gain understanding.")

- Trust in yourself and lean on your own understanding because this is the ultimate sign of maturity. (**Prov. 3:5-6** - "Trust in the LORD with all your heart and lean not on your own understanding; in all your ways acknowledge Him, and He will make your paths straight.")

- The Second Coming of Christ has already occurred or the early Disciples were mistaken about this, so forget it and get on with life. (**Matt. 25:13 -** "Therefore keep watch, because you do not know the day or the hour.")

- God loves sinners but hates sin so don't worry about being a sinner since all will be well in the long run. (**Matt. 7:23** - "Then I will tell them plainly, 'I never knew you. Away from Me, you evildoers!'")

- The Bible is not the only or even the ultimate Book where God has revealed Himself and His Will. (**Deut. 4:2** - "Do not add to what I command you and do not subtract from it, but keep the commands of the LORD your God that I give you." **Rev. 22:18-19** - "I warn everyone who hears the words of the prophecy of this book: If anyone adds anything to them, God will add to him the plagues described in this book. And if anyone takes words away from this book of prophecy, God will take away from him his share in the tree of life and in the holy city, which are described in this book.")

- God speaks in and through chosen people like the Mormon's Joseph Smith; the man behind the Watchtower, Charles Taze Russell; and Jim Jones, the founder of Jonestown who persuaded hundreds to commit suicide. (**Matt. 7:15** - "Watch out for false prophets. They come to you in sheep's clothing, but inwardly they are ferocious wolves.")

- Peace of mind is evil since it ignores all the evil that exists in this world, so true Christians should not seek peace. (**Ps. 34:14** - "Seek peace and pursue it." **Phil. 4: 4-7** - "Rejoice in the Lord always. I will say it again: Rejoice! Let your gentleness be evident to all. The Lord is near. Do not be anxious about anything, but in everything, by prayer and petition, with thanksgiving, present your requests to God. And the peace of God, which transcends all understanding, will guard your hearts and your minds in Christ Jesus.")

- God cannot be trusted to keep His Promises since circumstances will often cancel out those Promises. (**Num. 23:19** - "God is not a man, that He should lie, nor a son of man, that He should change His mind. Does He speak and then not act? Does He promise and not fulfill?")

- Many so-called rules and requirements of the Christian life are to be ignored and not taken seriously. (**Matt. 5:48** - "Be perfect, therefore, as your heavenly Father is perfect." **Gal. 6:7-8** - "Do not be deceived: God cannot be mocked. A man reaps what he sows. The one who sows to please his sinful nature, from that nature will reap destruction; the one who sows to please the Spirit, from the Spirit will reap eternal life.")

- Since the poor are always with us, it's okay to not care for the poor. (**Deut. 15:11** - "There will always be poor people in the land. Therefore I command you to be openhanded toward your brothers and toward the poor and needy in your land." **Matt. 25:40** - "The King will reply, 'I tell you the truth, whatever you did for one of the least of these brothers of Mine, you did for Me.'")

- Since we're all going to die, we might as well live this life to the fullest. (**John 11:26** - "Whoever lives and believes in Me will never die." **Gal. 6:7-8** - "Do not be deceived: God cannot be mocked. A man reaps what he sows. The one who sows to please his sinful nature, from that nature will reap destruction; the one who sows to please the Spirit, from the Spirit will reap eternal life.")

- Loving your body and taking good care of it is a sin and a sign of being self-centered and not Christ-centered. (**1 Cor. 6:19-20** - "Honor God with your body.")

- Since it will all burn anyway, it's okay to be foolish with money. (**1 Cor. 16:2** - "On the first day of every week, each one of you should set aside a sum of money in keeping with his income, saving it up, so that when I come no collections will have to be made." **1 Tim. 6:6-10** - "But godliness with contentment is great gain. For we brought nothing into the world, and we can take nothing out of it. But if we have food and clothing, we will be content with that. People who want to get rich fall into temptation and a trap and into many foolish and harmful desires that plunge men into ruin and destruction. For the love of money is a root of all kinds of evil. Some people, eager for money, have wandered from the faith and pierced themselves with many griefs.")

- People who claim to "hear from the Lord" are deluded. They are fanatics. They are nutty. They have gone off the deep end. They are to be avoided. (**1 Sam. 3:10** - "The LORD came and stood there, calling as at the other times, "Samuel! Samuel!" Then Samuel said, "Speak, for your servant is listening." **Rev. 3:19-20** - "Those whom I love I rebuke and discipline. So be earnest, and repent. Here I am! I stand at the door and knock. If anyone hears My voice and opens the door, I will come in and eat with him, and he with Me.")

- God loves everyone unconditionally. (**Mal. 1:3** - "Esau I have hated, and I have turned his mountains into a wasteland and left his inheritance to the desert jackals.")

What now?

It is much, much easier to discern Satan's lies if you know God's Holy Word. All kinds of crazy things are spoken today, but the Bible says you can test the spirits and know what is true and isn't true. First John 4:1-6 says, "Dear friends, do not believe every spirit, but test the spirits to see whether they are from God, because many false prophets have gone out into the world. This is how you can recognize the Spirit of God: Every spirit that acknowledges that Jesus Christ has come in the flesh is from God, but every spirit that does not acknowledge Jesus is not from God. This is the spirit of the antichrist, which you have heard is coming and even now is already in the world. You, dear children, are from God and have overcome them, because the one who is in you is greater than the one who is in the world. They are from the world and therefore speak from the viewpoint of the world, and the world listens to them. We are from God and whoever knows God listens to us; but whoever is not from God does not listen to us. This is how we recognize the Spirit of truth and the Spirit of falsehood." Simply said, you cannot trust a source that doesn't acknowledge the Lordship of Christ. Some preachers and teachers may say positive, seemingly-good things, but listen closely and see if they proclaim the Lordship of Christ or not. There you can find if their teaching is trustworthy, or if it is of Satan.

Any lie from Satan will deny the divinity and Lordship of Christ. People will tell you it's not necessary to believe in the

Virgin Birth, and the Physical Resurrection of Jesus. They'll say He was a good teacher. They'll say He was a prophet, and they may even call Him a miracle maker. But unless they claim Him as the Lord and God, they are believing and practicing a lie. Don't listen to them.

These deceived and other susceptible people will also disregard Scripture. They'll say the miracles in the Old and New Testaments are natural occurrences and that the Bible was written by mere men who spoke for themselves and not for God. Lots of sincere people espouse these teachings and beliefs, but they are also not worth listening to. Reject their thinking also.

As you read and believe Scripture, get to know as much as you can about Satan: how he thinks and why, what his limitations are, how you can defeat him, when will his kingdom end, etc. I'm not talking about being obsessed with Satan, but I'm talking about having a healthy understanding of who he is and what he does. I am convinced that the understanding God has given me on this subject is a major factor in enabling me to successfully cope with the myriad of plans the enemy has had to destroy my mind, heart, body and soul.

If Satan can be recognized and overcome through faith in and obedience to the God of the Bible, then you are well on your way to success, healing, victory, and overcoming sinful habits, etc. My heart goes out to people who are literally suffering due to attacks by the enemy and they are unaware of the course of the attacks. The Bible makes is very clear that if we resist Satan, he will flee (James 4:7). How can we resist him if we don't believe he exists and/or we are completely ignorant of his enormous powers? Again I say, and with great emphasis, recognition is extremely important!

Although Satan has enormous powers here on this earth, as the "ruler of this world," his power is limited. He is not to be feared, but acknowledged, understood and dealt with. That is why I (and you) must be totally surrendered to the Holy Spirit. The God of the Bible doesn't merely want me (and you) to be able to discern truth from lies. He wants me (and you) to step out in boldness and take His truth to a world attacked by Satan and dying from his lies. The God of the Bible wants me to go out, in His power and might, and display the Fruit of the Holy Spirit to all those I encounter. I am the hands and feet of Christ and as such, I need to walk in victory. In the next chapter, I'll explain how to walk in spiritual victory, exhibiting and enjoying what the Bible calls the Fruit of the Holy Spirit.

Chapter 5
Enjoying and Exhibiting the Fruit of the Spirit

The Spirit of the LORD will come upon you in power, and you will prophesy with Them; and you will be changed into a different person.
- 1 Samuel 10:6

The Spirit gives life; the flesh counts for nothing. The words I have spoken to you are spirit and they are life. - John 6:63

A great spiritual foundation goes beyond mere discernment of truth and lies. It includes a dynamic, growing relationship with the God of the Bible. In Biblical times, as well as today, Jesus calls people to "repent" (Matt. 4:17) and "follow Me" (Matt. 4:19). While early Christians enjoyed a close relationship with a physically present Jesus, His disciples today must, in faith, believe He is there. Today's disciple fellowships with an invisible God. (In Acts 2:33 it says that Jesus left this earth after His death and resurrection and ascended into Heaven, where He sits at the right hand of the Father.) Jesus knew it would be difficult for His followers to remain strong in Him if He wasn't physically there. So, Jesus made a promise to send His Spirit, a Counselor and Friend. He encouraged His followers by saying, "But the Counselor, the Holy Spirit, whom the Father will send in My name, will teach you all things and will remind you of everything I have said to you" (John 14:26). Jesus offers the same Holy Spirit to His followers today!

How does Jesus make this Counselor available to us? We must obey the God of the Bible. How many of you know someone who prayed the sinner's prayer a long time ago, but currently lives like he doesn't know Jesus? I imagine every reader of these words can name someone they know like that. These are people who give mental assent to being Christians but live un-righteously. They are *not* led by the Spirit of God. By disobeying God, even in the seemingly small stuff, the sinner refuses to listen to His Counsel. God only goes where He is invited and if a disobedient disciple chooses to obey an impulse other than God, then God will not force Himself and His will into the life of that person. Jesus says in John 14:23-24, "If anyone loves Me, he will obey My teaching. My Father will love him, and we will come to him and make Our home with him. He who does not love Me will not obey My teaching." If you want to enjoy great health in this life and in the life to come, obedience to God is essential because without obedience, not only will you be living in step with your sinful nature, but you'll miss out on the guidance and fellowship of the Holy Spirit.

Do you engage in sexual immorality; impurity and debauchery; idolatry and witchcraft; hatred, discord, jealousy, fits of rage, selfish ambition, dissensions, factions and envy; drunkenness, orgies, and the like? (Gal. 5: 19-21). If you do, you are disobeying God and are acting in line with a sinful nature. Jesus gives a stern warning to those who live like this: they will *not* inherit the kingdom of God (Gal. 5:22). In other words, your temporal and eternal health will suffer if you do these things.

The Fruit of the Spirit is listed in these verses (Gal. 5:22-25): "love, joy, peace, patience, kindness, goodness, faithfulness, gentleness and self-control. Against such things there is no law. Those who belong to Christ Jesus have crucified the sinful nature with its passions and desires. Since we live by the Spirit, let us keep in step with the Spirit." Living by the Spirit is a habit, a daily practice of listening to and obeying the voice of God. This fruit is for believers, those who have left their sins on the crucified Christ and have decided to follow God.

In September of 1947, I began my seminary training in a class of 39 male students at Fuller Theological Seminary in Pasadena, CA. The faculty and some of the students kept talking about the Holy Spirit being a real person and living in their minds/bodies/hearts/souls. I was confused. The liberal preaching/teaching to which I had been exposed after my father's home-going had not prepared me for this great truth.

I singled out fellow-student George Burch and simply asked, "What's this Holy Spirit all about?" He simply said, "Come with me" and led me to an empty classroom. He then said to me, "Let's both get on our knees and you ask God the same question you asked me." The result was almost instantaneous. Like John Wesley, I felt a "strange warmness" in my inner-being and an assurance of salvation that continues to grow to this day, plus a power to carry out God's daily assignments.

A Deeper Look

Galatians 5:22-25 is filled with meaning and promise for the Christian believer. The Greek word for "fruit" is singular, not plural. I suspect the God of the Bible is saying that *He* is the *one* tree that bears this fruit and not several trees. He, alone, is the One True God who offers these gifts to those who believe and obey. It is *one* fruit with nine expressions, or flavors. When we consume this fruit, it fills our lives with the stuff of God. It's nourishing, refreshing and delicious to taste.

The nine characteristics of the Fruit of the Spirit can be classified in three categories: inward attitudes, outward actions, and God-ward responses. The three inward attitudes are love, joy, and peace. These are attributes you experience within your own being. You can "feel" these attributes and you are strengthened by the Holy Spirit through them to be more like Christ. The next three characteristics are outward actions: patience, kindness, and goodness. You cannot manifest these attributes unless you are practicing them in conjunction with the prior three. These are attributes that others can witness and benefit from. This is when you begin to operate as the hands and feet of Christ, doing good works. The final three characteristics are God-ward responses: faithfulness, gentleness, and self-control. We do this for God and through God. All nine are the unmistakable marks of a Christian and are manifested in, by, and through the Holy Spirit.

The scripture goes on to say, "Against such things (meaning the Fruit of the Spirit), there is no law." In that time period, the Mosaic law demanded strict rules of conduct for the Israelites. There were rules for what types of activities you could do, when you do them and where you could do them. Some may have wondered where, when and under what circumstances they could practice the Fruit of the Spirit. Paul in his letter to the Galatians told them they could practice the Fruit anytime, anywhere and under any circumstances. There are no restrictions to exhibit the Fruit of the Spirit. Today, these attributes should, likewise, be practiced without restraint or fear of punishment from law bearers. The Fruit of the Spirit is always appropriate and always valid.

Paul also reminds the Galatians (and us today) that their sins are no longer their companions. Their sins have been crucified with Christ on the cross. Christ took the sins of the world, forever; so that everyone could be free, never to be enslaved by sin again. Paul is drawing a line in the sand and saying, your past life is behind you, and your new life in Christ is before you. Therefore, live by and through Christ's Holy Spirit.

In God's Strength

I have found that when I lose self-control and act un-Godly, I am consuming a different fruit, a counterfeit fruit. I'm not feasting on the Fruit of the Spirit. In my weakness, instead of turning to God for help, I temporarily allow the flesh (or my old man) to take over versus the Holy Spirit.

Thankfully, the solution is to not "try harder" or "press into God" but simply surrender to the Holy Spirit, Who blesses me with His fruit. It is a package deal, and when we surrender to the Holy Spirit, we are blessed with this fruit, which encompasses all nine expressions mentioned in Galatians 5:22-23.

Jesus again emphasizes the idea of surrender to the

leading and guiding of the Holy Spirit in an exchange He has with a crowd of people who had been looking for Him, "They asked Him, 'What must we do to do the works God requires?' Jesus answered, 'The work of God is this: to believe in the One He has sent'" (John 6: 28-29). Jesus takes away the emphasis on works and places it on belief. Romans 3:21-22 says, "But now a righteousness from God, apart from law, has been made known, to which the Law and the Prophets testify. This righteousness from God comes through faith in Jesus Christ to all who believe." The assumption is that if you believe in Jesus and His words, you'll obey and hence, clear out the static so the Holy Spirit can speak to you and fill you with His strength.

Again, to obey God you must be filled with God. Apart from listening to and believing in God, we can do works, but they amount to nothing. Isaiah 64:6 says, "All of us have become like one who is unclean, and all our righteous acts are like filthy rags." Good works cannot achieve a victorious life with great eternal health. They are an extension of a dynamic, living relationship with the God of the Bible. When you believe in God and surrender to Him, He fills you with His Holy Spirit, gives you His Fruit of the Spirit, and enables you to do those good works.

God shares an important truth on this subject in Zechariah 4:6 when He says "not by might, nor by power, but by My Spirit, says the Lord Almighty." I believe He is saying the Christian life begins in and by the Holy Spirit (new birth = born again) and can only be sustained in, by, and through the Holy Spirit.

This lifestyle of living and walking by and through the Holy Spirit is not new. It's not just a New Testament phenomenon. The Old Testament prophets listened to and recorded the words of Holy Spirit. Micah writes in 3:8, "I am filled with power, with the Spirit of the LORD, and with justice and might, to declare to Jacob his transgression, to Israel his sin."

Jesus, Himself, needed the Holy Spirit. Luke 3:21-23 says, "And as He was praying, heaven was opened and the Holy Spirit descended on Him in bodily form like a dove. And a voice came from heaven: 'You are My Son, whom I love; with You I am well pleased.'" God from Heaven encouraged and empowered Jesus to do His ministry on earth by giving Him the Holy Spirit. God in Heaven waits to encourage and empower you, too, by giving you His Holy Spirit today. It starts with faith.

If you don't have faith and try to be good on your own strength, you'll fail. Doing good and displaying the Fruit of the Spirit is difficult if you are trying to do it in your own strength. In fact, you can't. The key is to surrender to God and let Him live His life through you. Philippians 4:13 says, "You can do everything through Him Who gives you strength."

In another verse, Peter also exhorts others to use the strength of God. 1 Peter 4:11 says, "If anyone speaks, he should do it as one speaking the very words of God. If anyone serves, he should do it with the *strength God provides*, so that in all things God may be praised through Jesus Christ. To Him be the glory and the power for ever and ever. Amen." This strength is made available to us through belief in God, and trusting in the Holy Spirit.

I've often compared the Christian life to a boat where the rower tries to use the oars to propel the boat versus using the power motor. Supernatural power is not available by mustering it with our own will power; it's only available when the Holy Spirit is allowed to come into our minds, hearts, souls, and bodies through faith.

Satan can provide an unbeliever with one or more of the attributes listed in Galatians 5:22-23 but not the "package deal." In other words, Satan can give a man patience and persuade him that he is right with God and need not fear about the future of his soul. However, Satan cannot give a man *all* the fruit of the Spirit, because Satan's sole objective is to lie, kill, steal and destroy. If he can give you one or two attributes of the Fruit of the Spirit to deceive you and your relationship with God, then He will. But, he wouldn't want, nor is he able to give you all of them because that would be too much of a blessing, and Satan has no power to be that good.

Beware of Counterfeit Fruit

Have you ever seen wax or plastic fruit sitting in a bowl at someone's home? It may look real but if you pick it up and begin to eat it, you will soon realize that you are dealing with counterfeit fruit. Your natural response is to spit it out and refuse to eat it. So should your response be if you try to ingest counterfeit Fruit of the Spirit.

Here are some counterfeit fruits: resignation, unease, sniping, irritability, selfishness, and meanness. These are not exactly opposites of the Fruit of the Spirit, but they miss the mark of what God really wants you to experience. Now read these opposites, attributes that completely miss the mark: hate, sadness, turmoil, impatience, unkindness, evil, unfaithfulness, cruelty, and lack of self-control.

Unfortunately, many believers have accepted these false fruits and have justified consuming them by saying, "God is holding out on me. This is the best I can find in this life."

This lie from Satan has given poor health to millions. God wants to give you better fruit and you can have better if you would spit out the false fruit, reach out in faith to the God Who wants to fill you with His Spirit, obey Him, and accept His real, delicious, nourishing Fruit of the Spirit. If you are missing out on some of the Fruit of the Spirit, make an appeal to the God of the Bible. Ask God to give you *all* the fruit, and ask Him to show you where you have erred if you are not having access to or enjoying *all* the Fruit of the Spirit. God is faithful and will respond to a humble prayer like this.

You may be tempted to be jealous of unbelievers who seem to enjoy many attributes of the Fruit of the Spirit. But watch these same people when adversity strikes. For some, it's easy to be a fair-weather, joyful, kind person. But when the storms of life hit, they'll buckle and resort to exhibiting counterfeit fruits.

It has been reported that the notorious gangster, Al Capone, established a reputation in San Quentin for being very kind, considerate, humble, thoughtful, patient, gentle, etc., when in fact it was known that he personally ordered the torture and execution of hundreds of people who opposed his racketeering and other crimes. Perhaps he turned to God in prison and received the Fruit of the Spirit. But, history suggests a different fate. After he was convicted and imprisoned on charges of tax evasion, he eventually went mad. Unable to access life-saving drugs, the symptoms of his syphilis returned and he eventually died after an apoplectic stroke, pneumonia and cardiac arrest. Great health from God evaded Al Capone and he died a fairly young man.

Another danger to watch out for is claiming you "hear" a Word from the Holy Spirit, but it's contrary to God's written Word, the Holy Bible. Such a false word might be, "God told me I could commit adultery with another woman." Another lie might be, "God said it was okay for me to steal these things because I need them for my business to stay alive." If you think God is telling you to do something contrary to what He already said in His Word, beware. (Exod. 12:14 says, "You shall not commit adultery." Exod. 20:15 says, "You shall not steal.") God's spoken and written Word will always agree.

The Greek work "logos" refers to the written word of God, while the Greek word "rhema" refers to the spoken word of God. The written Word is given to us via the Bible while the spoken is given via the Holy Spirit. The God of the Bible also speaks through faithful servants who speak under the power and leadership of the Holy Spirit (such as preachers, pastors, evangelists, Bible teachers, etc.) These two "Words" of God must always agree and not contradict each other. If you hear a spoken word from a preacher that is contrary to the written Word of God, it is not from God and is not to be followed. If you get a "hunch" in your Spirit and it is contrary to the Word of God, it is not from God and is not to be followed.

If you immerse yourself into the Word of God, you'll learn to discern if a spoken Word is from the God of the Bible or not. You can also test and see if those "hunches" you have are from the Holy Spirit, or from somewhere or someone else. Immersing yourself in God's Word will also make it easier for God to remind you of His promises when you need to hear them. He'll "quicken" or remind you of life-giving Words that you can apply throughout your day. John 6:63 says, "The Spirit gives life; the flesh counts for nothing. The words I have spoken to you are spirit and they are life." Talk about great health!

The Fruits in My Life

At the prompting of the Holy Spirit, I accepted Jesus Christ as my Lord and Savior, and then began to daily learn lessons from Him, which still occur today. I learned that it took a supernatural Holy Spirit within to produce a supernatural life without. Before that experience, I was relying too much on my own understanding and on my own flesh. What a difference in everyday life to realize I had this supernatural Person actually living inside me, wanting me to know Him, to use Him, to trust Him, to learn from Him. For some reason, I had not thought of the Holy Spirit as an actual Person but simply a non-entity, a thing, a life-less power that came with accepting Jesus Christ as Lord and Savior. To this day I cannot explain in words how the God of the Bible can be One and yet manifest Himself in Three Persons (a.k.a the Holy Trinity) but I am so very grateful that the God of the Bible exists this way. I don't feel I need to understand the complexity of His nature, but all I have to do is simply believe and accept Him, and put into practice what He tells me (obey Him). This simple plan has benefited me all the days of my life.

God taught me one lesson about the Holy Spirit by reminding me of a story about a European immigrant. Years ago, before airplanes, this man felt led of the Holy Spirit to come to the United States and pursue opportunities to make a good living. He figured he could make enough money in the U.S. that he could send money to his family and they could likewise take an ocean liner and join him in this great land of opportunity. His funds were greatly limited but he managed to save enough money to purchase a ticket for the trip over to the U.S. Never having been on the ocean, he assumed food costs were extra so his wife prepared a box of long-lasting food items designed to sustain him on the long trip across the Atlantic Ocean. Imagine his surprise, when upon arriving in New York, he discovered that the ticket price also included three meals a day in the ship's dining room!

I felt exactly like that when I realized at age 25, that upon becoming a Christian at age 9, I was entitled to *all* the fruit of the Holy Spirit. I had not been taking full advantage of all the entitlements that had come with accepting Jesus Christ as Lord and Savior. Thankfully, unlike the immigrant who had completed his voyage, I realized I had plenty of time left on my voyage. As long as I had years left in my life here on earth, I had access to God's power through the Holy Spirit. Therefore, for many years now, my life has been guided and empowered by the Holy Spirit. And the Holy Spirit has convinced me that the Bible *is* the Word of God and can be trusted fully. The Holy Spirit also has convinced me that Jesus Christ is *all He claimed to be.* Those two truths have benefited me immeasurably and have contributed mightily to my great health.

I am reminded in Hebrews 11:6 that God "rewards those who earnestly seek Him." As I seek after God and believe in Him, I want to give Him all praise, glory, honor, and credit for any benefit that I receive. In all actuality, I deserve eternal hell, but God in His mercy, listened to my cry for mercy and not only saved me from my sin, but gave me the Fruit of His Spirit. My great health is not my own doing, even though I do my best to take care of my body, but it is the result of nearly 80 years of faith and trust in God.

I do not take this gift of great health for granted. God certainly has the right, at any time, to take not only my great health away from me, but also the Fruit of His Spirit (especially if I decide to disobey Him!) Deuteronomy 6:13-

19 makes it very clear that God is a jealous God and He insists on being #1 in our lives. He will not share His Throne with anyone or anything else. If I do not put Him as #1, His anger will "burn against me" and He will "destroy me from the face of the earth" (Deut. 6:15). This is a powerful and fearful promise that still applies today because "He is the same God yesterday, today, and forever. He has not changed" (Heb. 3:8).

Even though I try to be a faithful disciple, I sometime fall short of exhibiting one or more of the attributes of the Fruit of the Spirit. Even though I am born again by a work of the Holy Spirit and not the flesh, I am still living in a body of flesh, which has its own desires contrary to the Spirit and will of God. The Apostle Paul understood this and said, "For in my inner being I delight in God's law; but I see another law at work in the members of my body, waging war against the law of my mind and making me a prisoner of the law of sin at work with my members" (Rom. 7: 22, 23). Woefully, this is a wretched state, but like Paul, I also give thanks to the solution to this dilemma. "Thanks be to God – through Jesus Christ our Lord!" (Rom. 7:25)

Though I may fail, Christ and His shed blood covers over my sin. If I continue to believe Christ for His atoning work in the forgiveness of my sins and if I continue to believe that Christ is making His Holy Spirit available to me, I can live a life controlled by the Spirit, which is "life and peace" (Rom. 8:6). With the Holy Spirit living in me, I press forward in faith like the Apostle Paul, who says in Philippians 3:12-14, "I press on to take hold of that for which Christ Jesus took hold of me. Brothers, I do not consider myself yet to have taken hold of it. But one thing I do: Forgetting what is behind and straining toward what is ahead, I press on toward the goal to win the prize for which God has called me heavenward in Christ Jesus." Hence, I strive for perfection, which Jesus also commands in Matthew 5:48. Thankfully, I know that God is here to forgive me if I repent, ask for His forgiveness, and seek His face when I fail.

Furthermore, the more I trust in and lean on Jesus, the more strength I receive from the Holy Spirit to obey and follow Him. As I receive, practice, and appreciate the gift of the Fruit of the Holy Spirit, I also enjoy great health. (I've not had perfect health, but God has given me an ability to give Him thanks in all things. And that has gotten me through good times and bad.) Those who reject the God of the Bible and those who practice the opposite of the Fruit of the Spirit often have all kinds of physical, mental, spiritual, and emotional problems. Hate and the inability to forgive and unfaithfulness can destroy you.

If you fear losing your faith in God, take comfort in this verse from Philippians 1:6, "being confident of this, that He who began a good work in you will carry it on to completion until the day of Christ Jesus." God loves to bless, guide and protect those who would place their faith in Him. He loves to offer His Fruit of the Spirit to all who would dare to believe.

God is so good. He wants to give you His Holy Spirit to have a successful, great life. He has opened up all of who He is for your benefit. When you have a strong spiritual foundation, the rest of your life can rest assured that your base is strong. In the next section, ***Layer Two: Physical Health***, I'll write about how to gain and keep great physical health. You'll read how physical health and spiritual health are interconnected, and how physical health can be enhanced by a dynamic, growing relationship with the Living God of the Bible.

Layer Two: Physical Health

Chapter 6
Eating (and Drinking) Right

Consider the ravens: They do not sow or reap, they have no storeroom or barn; yet God feeds them. And how much more valuable you are than birds! - Luke 12:24

I am the bread of life: he that cometh to Me shall never hunger; and he that believeth in Me shall never thirst. - John 6:35

Since the beginning of time, God has been concerned about what we humans put into our mouths. Even before Eve was created, the very first words that God spoke to Adam were about food. God said in Genesis 2:16 -17, "You are free to eat from any tree in the garden; but you must not eat from the tree of the knowledge of good and evil, for when you eat of it you will surely die." With that command, God gave man enormous gastronomic freedom. God said he could eat from *any* tree but one. That means hundreds, thousands, perhaps millions of possibilities. *Everything* in the garden was good to eat, except for the fruit from that one tree.

With His command, God was saying to man, "Obedience to Me is more important than your appetites and cravings."

God wanted man to freely choose to obey Him. He didn't want to make a robot that would automatically obey, mimicking pre-programmed commands. God wanted a creation with free-will that would turn to God and obey Him on his own volition. Hence, the tree of the knowledge of good and evil was put in the garden as a test to see if Adam would obey God or not. Unfortunately, we all know the end of that story: Adam and Eve ate of the fruit and were banished from the Garden because of their sin.

Is the food you are eating drawing you closer to God, or pulling you away from Him? Face it. We, like Adam, have all gone astray and eaten wrongfully. We've all over-eaten, under-eaten, eaten foods that are too fatty, too sugary, too filled with cancer-causing preservatives, or just plain imbalanced. We've displeased God with the way we have treated our bodies.

Just because we may have displeased God with our sins of consumption, doesn't mean we have to permanently live in sin as a bad eater. There is a better way. The God of the Bible made a way to save Adam from his sins and He also made a way to save you from your sins through Christ. 1 Corinthians 6:19-20 says, "Do you not know that your body is a temple of the Holy Spirit, Who is in you, Whom you have received from God? You are not your own; you were bought at a price. Therefore honor God with your body." These Bible verses were written to the Corinthians about abstaining from sexual immorality, but I believe it can equally apply to us today about abstaining from poor eating habits.

So how do you honor God with your eating and in so doing give yourself the best chance for great health? I think an important first step is to recognize and then overcome the obstacles that have prevented you from changing your diet sooner. Below are common lies (or excuses) that people use to justify their poor eating habits. If you discover that you too have believed these lies, why not repent of them today?

Common Lies about Poor Eating Habits

Lie #1: I'm too tired to prepare healthy foods.

In today's hurried society, you may be tempted to skip eating well for the quick and easy fast-food alternative. Resist this urge. If you are so tired from work that you abuse your body with junk food, then you need to get a new job! Life is too short and your body is too important to God for you to abuse it. Living a stress-filled life is no life at all and it's not a life God wants for you. You may not be able to change your job or the amount of stress in your life right away. Some adjustments over time are required for true change. But don't use your work as an excuse for poor eating.

Lie #2: My patterns or poor eating habits are ingrained. I cannot change.

Unless you have a very rare disease where you always have feelings of hunger, you *can* control the amount of food you put into your body. And *everybody* can control the type of food they consume. In a world full of accidents and surprises, it's refreshing that there is one thing that we can control which will shape our health destiny: our diet. The God of the Bible has given you a fantastic gift called free will. Exercise it! Use it! Take advantage of it! You are not controlled by your appetites. Changing your diet and/

or controlling your diet may be difficult for a time, but it will help you stay healthy. Do whatever it takes to free yourself from the ties that bind you and hold you back from eating well.

I think every besetting, long-standing food-addiction has a demonic component to it. James 4:7 says, "Submit yourselves, then, to God. Resist the devil, and he will flee from you." Believe it or not, after awhile, abnormal cravings can and will disappear when you resist them. Whether or not your food problems have a demonic component to them, God can deliver you from your food addictions and bad habits. If your problems are extreme, you may need to check into a "fat" camp where, for a time, you are "forced" to eat what they give you. This time may be unpleasant and difficult, but if you are "re-trained" with good eating habits, you can emerge stronger, more in control of yourself, and now eating and drinking better. Less extreme eating abnormalities may only require a food coach, an accountability partner, or a group like Weight Watchers. But help is available. Take advantage of it.

Lie #3: I don't have access to healthy foods.

If you live in America, you *do* have access to healthy foods. Every town may not have a health food store, but every town has a grocery store and every grocery store now has fresh produce (fruits and vegetables), whole grain breads, organic foods, fat-free, sugar-free and nutritious foods of every kind. (Personally, I'm leery of fat-free and sugar-free because that often means that the food has unnatural, health-risky ingredients in them like preservatives, food colors, and other cancer-causing agents, etc.) Although junk foods abound, healthier foods are also prevalent. The last 20 to 40 years has brought about a boom in health-conscious eating. You can find healthy foods to eat. They are as close to you as your grocery store.

Lie #4: Healthy (or Organic) foods are too expensive.

This lie is actually partially true. Go into any organic food aisle or health food store, and you'll see prices for products that are higher than their "non-organic," "non-healthy" alternatives. If you are going to totally commit yourself to the ultra-healthy lifestyle and shop exclusively at health food stores, you will probably pay a premium for it. Thankfully, you do not have to shop at health food stores or buy organic to be healthy.

A study published in June 2009 in the *American Journal of Clinical Nutrition* says that conventional foods are just as nutritious as organic foods.[1] This is great news for all who want to eat nutritious food but don't want to pay the premium price for organic foods. You *can* find healthy equivalent foods at your normal, local grocery store that will offer you the same nutritional value as the so-called "healthier" organic foods, and they'll be a lot less expensive.

Once you have recognized and owned up to the lies that have held you back from eating well, your next step is to develop good eating habits and finding family and friends that will help keep you on track.

1 Corinthians 15:33 says, "Do not be misled: Bad company corrupts good character." If your buddies are into chips, cheese and beer and being couch potatoes, it

will be much, much harder for you to eat right than if you have supportive friends. Granted, you may only hang-out with your friends once or twice a week, so it's all the more important to have your family, those you are with more often than not, to know and respect your dietary needs and support you as you are trying to not only eat better, but develop a healthier lifestyle.

If you are married, your spouse will play a key role in how, what, where, why and when you will eat. Your spouse can exert tremendous power over you with your diet. If you have a spouse who is supportive of your dietary goals, your marriage will not only be strengthened, but together you can build a strong force against those other forces that say you should not eat healthy. I'm proud to say I am married to the world's best partner when it comes to planning meals. My beloved wife, Margaret Ann, sees to it that our diet includes the proper and daily requirements of vitamins, protein, carbohydrates, etc., in our three daily meals. She very carefully selects fruits, vegetables, meats, and liquids that have proven in the past to make us and keep us healthy.

If you are trying to change your diet, insist your spouse help you along the way. His or her help is crucial and you'll both benefit from eating well. Messages abound that say, "Try this cake. Sample this delicious food. Enjoy this delectable." The advertisers don't tell you what the wrapper (by law) reveals: all the calories, fat-content and cancer-causing preservatives the processed food contains. With a strong supportive spouse, you can reject these messages and learn to discern which foods are better for you than others. In time, those advertising messages won't even be a temptation.

The joke goes, "The best way to avoid temptation is to

give in to it." Nonsense! Temptation is best circumvented when that certain food ceases to be tempting. (Another joke says, "Nothing tastes as good as thin feels." This is closer to the truth and closer to the point I am trying to make.) Temptations are severely reduced or eliminated when you develop a strong affinity for the opposite of the temptation. You become so desirous of healthy food and healthy living that the allure of junk food vanishes. If you yield your life over to the Lordship of Christ, and you walk in His Spirit, you already have the tools to resist and reduce temptation and to develop a new lifestyle.

While it is easy to develop bad habits (because they don't really require sacrifice or an act of the will), it's a little harder to develop good eating habits. But practice makes perfect and good habits soon become second nature. You'll eventually develop a habit of buying and eating healthier foods, and your automatic response will be to grab a piece of fruit versus a candy bar or bag of chips. In time, a habit will develop into a lifestyle. You will not need to resist temptation because your temptations or cravings for bad food will disappear if not diminish significantly.

My Eating Journey

As I said in the introduction, I am not a nutritionist, nor a medical specialist. I only know that eating (and drinking) right have served me well, and has allowed me to serve and obey my God at a much higher level than if I had not eaten right. The key word to what I eat and drink is "balance." I try not to overeat or under-eat. My beloved wife is tops when it comes to planning meals and I try to follow her advice and eat and drink what she puts before me.

I eat plenty of fresh vegetables and fruits, meats such as fish, turkey, chicken, beef, and pork, all cooked to perfection. I do not eat a lot of fried foods. I eat fresh eggs two or three times a week, usually soft-boiled, and homemade bread, at which my wife excels. I drink fresh juices such as orange, carrot, grapefruit, grape, and cran-raspberry (a combo of cranberry juice and various berries). I drink plenty of water. (I probably drink a half-gallon of liquids each day.) I drink a quart or more of milk each day, usually 2%, and I usually drink milk with each meal, especially lunch and dinner. Although I love dessert and have a little dessert usually after lunch and dinner, I try not to overdo this. I weigh myself daily and keep my weight below 200 pounds (At 6 feet 2 and one-half inches tall, I keep myself fit and lean.). I eat meals on schedule. Breakfast is at 5:45 A.M., lunch at 11 A.M. (followed by 2 hour nap), and dinner is at 5:30 P.M. I really hate to get off this schedule but at times it becomes necessary. For snacking, I eat half a fresh apple daily around 5 P.M. and I eat two prunes daily before breakfast. I also drink two cups of warm water when I get up in the morning, which also helps greatly with bowel movements. We have two orange trees, one lemon tree, one fig tree and these trees provide fresh fruit for us several months out of the year.

I also take daily food supplements such as one Multi-Vitamin Multi-Mineral Supplement, especially formulated for adults 50 and over, from A to Zinc. I also take one 81 mg Aspirin. (This is on doctor's orders, and it helps keep my blood thin, and prevents heart attack.) I also use Fish Oil, which reduces risk of coronary heart disease. And, I take one dose of Sea Kelp, a natural source of mineral iodine which is an essential component of the thyroid hormone that plays a role in growth, development, and metabolic rate. I consume garlic and parsley for a healthy heart and it also helps control cholesterol. One Cider-Vinegar is great and it's a healthy supplement for healthy fitness and nutrition, and one Glucosamine Sulfate and MSM, which is derived from shellfish and helps control arthritis, bursitis, etc.

I eat one dose of Queen Bee Royal Jelly, made by Bee Alive, Inc. Queen Bee Royal Jelly is rich in vitamins and protein; it is a creamy substance formed by glands in the heads of young worker bees. The workers produce this for the Queen Bee and she lives for five years or so. Neither worker bees nor drone bees eat this Royal Jelly and they live only six weeks or so. I've been taking this vitamin for several years and swear by it. It has really helped me in several ways (such as boosting my energy level, helping me feel great, etc.).

I also take one Aleve or two Ibuprofens daily to help ease back pain due to the two lowest vertebral discs being completely gone, creating a bone on bone situation in my lower back. Each morning, I also put on my back either Ben Gay, Aspercreme, or a Pain Relieving Back Patch. These products that I use and consume have kept me going all these years. They may or may not be right for you. Consult your doctor before starting a new diet, or dietary supplement program.

Functional Eater

Since I believe I was made by God for God's purposes, my body belongs to Him. I eat and drink to fuel myself for His purposes. As I keep this in mind, I become very conscious on a daily basis of what I eat and drink and how much I eat and drink. A fellow Christian friend of mine years ago described himself as a "functional eater." He went on to say he tried to only put in his mouth food and drink that would enable him to "function efficiently" for his wonderful Creator. He says he eats to live, and does not live to eat. He also realizes that satisfying the lusts of the flesh in gluttonous eating not only displeases God, it takes away from his "functionality" or effectiveness for God and His Kingdom. I like this thinking and agree.

God gave "functional" food to the Israelites in the desert. The Bible calls this food "Manna." In the book of Exodus, the Israelites led by Moses were traveling to the "promised land" after being released from slavery in Egypt. Though these Israelites were impatient and often rebellious, God provided food for them in the dry, arid desert. Exodus 11:7-9 says, "The manna was like coriander seed and looked like resin. The people went around gathering it, and then ground it in a handmill or crushed it in a mortar. They cooked it in a pot or made it into cakes. And it tasted like something made with olive oil. When the dew settled on the camp at night, the manna also came down." Scriptures go on to say in Exodus 16:35, "The Israelites ate manna forty years, until they came to a land that was settled; they ate manna until they reached the border of Canaan." This foodstuff (along with quail, which God also provided for protein) sustained the Israelites for forty years and made them able to function and move forward, until their journey was complete.

Today, your "functional" food need not be as bland as manna, but the food lessons of Exodus and Numbers are the same. The lessons are not about the flavor or variety of

God's functional food, but about God's provision. He is our provider and can provide for our daily sustenance in even the most scarce, driest conditions. God provides all our food needs in order for us to "function" and do His will. You were made by Him for Him and He feeds you for His purposes.

I really like that philosophy, though I admit it is hard to always follow through. I admit I love to eat and sometimes I eat things that are not necessarily good for me (like rich desserts, etc.). But that leads me to my next point and that is about moderation.

Everything in Moderation

Remember those first words that God gave Adam in Genesis 2? "You are free to eat from any tree in the garden." One lesson I take away from this is that God approves of a diet that includes a lot of foods, more foods than you might think. Who do you think created the cocoa plant, the coffee plant, the sugar cane, and the chicken egg? The God of the Bible, that's Who! Chocolate, coffee, sugar and eggs have all gotten a bad wrap in the health press. (Ironically, there has been, of late, more positive press on these so-called bad foods.) But if you eat them in a level that isn't gluttonous, you can eat them. God approves.

Name one of the healthiest foods imaginable. Broccoli? Apples? Blueberries? Carrots? Imagine if you ate these foods to excess. At the very least, you'd get a stomach ache. At most, you may develop health problems because you would have deficiencies in nutrients these foods do not provide. Anything in excess is bad for you.

What about tobacco and alcohol? Do I use those products

in moderation? I do not, nor do I recommend that you use them either. While I see no reason to drink hard liquor or beer, there are some studies that suggest a little red wine may be good for you. But there is an alternative to red wine. Dr. Peter Gott, writing an advice column in the *Ventura County Star* says, "Studies have indicated that resveratrol and other antioxidants in red wine might prevent heart disease and arterial damage, while increasing levels of good cholesterol. Resveratrol is believed to be the main ingredient in wine that keeps blood vessels healthy and prevents blood clots; however, most reported research has been performed on animals, not humans. Those studies also revealed testing on mice were positive for the prevention of diabetes and obesity, both strong risk factors for heart disease. Resveratol can also be found in cranberries, blueberries, and peanuts. It is estimated that for a person to reap the same full benefits of resveratol that mice do, an individual will have to consume between 100 and 1,000 bottles of red wine daily."[3] Since I can receive the same health benefits from other foods as I do from red wine, I abstain. Furthermore, the risks I may face by consuming red wine (drunkenness, bad witness to others, etc.) far outweigh any benefits I might receive through its consumption.

Frankly, if I were to lean on my own understanding, I would indulge in both smoking and drinking - in moderation of course. But God makes it very clear that I am not to lean on my own understanding but upon His, and every time I commit these two items to Him in prayer, I get the same answer, which is, "No, don't indulge." How do I know I'm hearing from God Himself? I don't *know* but I *have* faith, and if I err, I err on the side of caution and restraint.

The God of the Bible asks us to be sober. Proverbs 23:21

says, "Drunkards and gluttons become poor, and drowsiness clothes them in rags." 1 Corinthians 6:10 warns that drunkards will not inherit the Kingdom of God. Ephesians 5:18 says what our goal should be: "Do not get drunk on wine, which leads to debauchery. Instead, be filled with the Spirit." While it may be permissible for me to consume wine in moderation, I choose instead to be filled with the Spirit. That way, I won't miss out on anything God wants to offer me.

In Conclusion

The old adage "You are what you eat" is true. Your health, spiritual, mental, emotional, and physical, can be measured by what you subject your body too, and what you put into it. Just as you don't want bad counsel, you don't want bad food. Bad foods make the mind and the body soft. The God of the Bible equips our minds and bodies to do different tasks, regardless if these jobs are menial or challenging, mental or physical. No matter what job God has given us to do, we need to keep our minds and bodies functioning by eating the proper food. Quality-in means quality-out.

I don't wish to overestimate or underestimate the importance of a good daily diet but I will say I think it is impossible to enjoy excellent health without it. People have lived and thrived on high-protein, high-fat diets (the Inuit of Greenland); on low-protein, high-carb diets (the indigenous peoples of southern Africa); on diets high in raw milk and cream (the people of the Loetschental Valley in Switzerland); diets high in saturated fat (the Trobriand Islanders), and even on diets in which animal blood is considered a staple (the Massai of Kenya and Tanzania). And folks have thrived on these diets without the ravages of degenerative diseases that are so epidemic in modern American life—heart disease, diabetes, obesity, neurodegenerative diseases, osteoporosis and cancer. The only thing these diets have in common is that they're all based on whole foods with minimal processing.[2]

Many people have it stuck in their minds that everything that tastes good is bad for you and everything that tastes bad is good for you. This is also nonsense! Get that out of your mind right away. There are more recipes available now than ever that celebrate flavor and satisfaction while using fresh, wholesome, tasty ingredients. The varieties of healthy, delicious salad, casserole, sauce, side dish and entrée recipes are a lot of fun to read and explore. And cooking or assembling new recipes is a fun activity you can do alone or with your spouse. The results are something you can be proud of and are something you can share with others. Who knows? You may be a gourmet chef just waiting to come out of your shell. If you try new recipes, your family, friends, church congregation or even strangers can benefit from the fruits of your labor! Eating right needn't be drudgery, but a fun social activity that many can enjoy.

Footnotes

1. http://www.ajcn.org/misc/release1.shtml#dang.
2. http://health.msn.com/nutrition/articlepage.aspx?cp-documentid=100241585>1=31036.
3. Gott, Dr. Peter, "Is Red Win Good for the Heart, and How Much?" *Ventura County Star*, September 5, 2009.

Chapter 7
Exercise Each and Every Day

Do you not know that in a race all the runners run, but only one gets the prize? Run in such a way as to get the prize. Everyone who competes in the games goes into strict training. They do it to get a crown that will not last; but we do it to get a crown that will last forever. Therefore I do not run like a man running aimlessly; I do not fight like a man beating the air. No, I beat my body and make it my slave so that after I have preached to others, I myself will not be disqualified for the prize. - 1 Corinthians 9:24-27

In the early days of history, man walked everywhere he had to go. Few had the luxury of a horse or a horse drawn carriage or wagon. The mostly widely used mode of transportation was foot power-walking. Because mankind needed to exert energy as a necessity for living, many people were lean and physically fit. Obesity was reserved for the infirm or the elderly. Walking meant fitness, and organized, recreational exercise was held only at rare, special events.

Then in the 8th century, B.C. (Before Christ), athletic competitions were taken to a new level of organization.

Several of the city-states of Ancient Greece near Olympia banded together to compete against each other. Included in the games were combat events, a pentathlon, boxing, wrestling, equestrian events, and running. Around 400 A.D., after the Romans outlawed pagan cults and destroyed Greek temples, the Olympic Games ended.

During this Olympic period, some of the Old Testament was written and all of the New Testament was recorded. No doubt, many of the writers that God used to create these books of the Bible knew about organized athletic competition. The word "run" (in the context of moving swiftly on your feet) is listed nearly 100 times in the Bible and the word "runner" twice. "Race," as in moving your feet swiftly to win a competition, is listed ten times. "Wrestle," as in grappling, is listed twice, as in the time Jacob wrestled a man of God (Genesis 32).

Even when the Bible isn't talking about recreational or competitive running, its use of the word "run" always includes a spiritual lesson. In Genesis 19, when Sodom and Gomorrah are about to be destroyed for their wickedness, Lot appeals to God in verse 20 and he says, "Look, here is a town near enough to *run* to, and it is small. Let me flee to it - it is very small, isn't it? Then my life will be spared." In this context, Lot talks about running as a means to preserving his life.

Contrary to what you might think, having a body and taking care of it is a very holy and Biblical thing to do. Some sects and religious orders deny the body (and think the soul and spirit are the only things in life that matter) and other sects abuse the body (and practice self-flagellation or self-mutilation). The God of the Bible created matter, including human bodies, and He called us "good." He also came to earth as the God-man Jesus and lived among us, proving that He was not beneath appearing in human flesh, but rather, He respected who we are and what He had created to live as one of us.

Having a body is good. For now, we live in a material world and we need our material body to do the work of God. Taking care of your body is essential if you are to fully function at top performance for the purposes and use of God. In addition to eating right, having strong bones and muscles, a good cardio-vascular system and flexible joints obtained through exercise, will equip you to do what God wants you to do.

America is more obese now than it has ever been. Colleagues at San Francisco General Hospital and Columbia University, estimate that by 2020, as many as 44% of American women and 37% of men, at age 35, will be obese - obese and, therefore, ill.[1] Preventable diseases like early onset Type 2 Diabetes and coronary disease can be prevented with exercise. Television, internet, video games, office jobs, the safety and comfort of your own home, and other factors contribute to a sedentary lifestyle, which many people easily fall into today. Unless you are physically unable to exercise, there's no good reason why you shouldn't. Below are some of the common lies today that people say about not exercising. After each lie, I've also included my rebuttal. I hope I can encourage you to successfully resist these lies and live life anew. You can do it!

Common Lies about Poor Exercise Habits

Lie #1: I'm too tired (or too busy) to exercise.

It's true. We live in a busy, fast-paced world. Meetings, school boards, volunteer, community service, family obligations, and work deadlines all take us away from being physically active. At the end of the work day, many are too tired and merely want to "crash on the couch." It's hard just to stay alive. Living becomes surviving. There is a better way.

This is when time-management comes into play. If your life is out of balance, something has to give. If your life is causing you utter exhaustion, then you need to change your life. There may be brief moments where you have to concentrate more fully on outside activities (such as a project with a deadline), but living day-after-day, week-after-week, month-after-month, and year-after-year where it's rush-rush-rush all the time, that is not God's best. It's a quick track to burnout, or worse, irreparable damage to your health. You can live a life in balance.

Right now, slow down. Close your eyes and take a deep breath. Go ahead and do it. There. Now, think about all the things you are doing to fill your days and see if there is anything which immediately comes to mind that you can drop or cut back on. Is everything you do really essential? If you can't think of anything, pray and ask the Holy Spirit to show you how to prioritize your day. Ask the Holy Spirit to show you how to live. The God of the Bible doesn't want you burned out. He wants you to be energetic and accessible.

Consider exercising at the beginning of the morning, before your day gets hectic. If you need to listen to audio reports or watch video footage for work, consider installing a treadmill near your TV, Stereo or A/V equipment. (Walking is such an easy and low-impact exercise that I recommend it to everyone.) See if your workplace has a fitness or health program associated with its health care package, and take advantage of it. Nothing can be more fun than taking your competitive drive at work and channeling it into physical competition with your work associates. Consider tennis, racquetball, swimming, golf or other competitive sports with your work associates. Even weight training with another can be fun.

If you are retired, you have even less of an excuse. You probably have a lot more free time than the fellow who works full-time. Go ahead and find a neighbor, family member, or church member, and discover a new sport together. Present goals and challenges to each other and work together to meet those goals. When you work out with someone else, you'll strengthen your relationship and help each other achieve your goals.

Lie #2: I've never exercised, so why should I start?

A body in motion stays in motion and a body at rest tends to stay at rest. If you keep telling yourself that you don't need exercise, you'll never get off your couch. You must reach a point where the benefits and joys (and sometimes necessity) of exercise outweigh the pains and the old-standby, "I don't feel like it." You may never feel like it, especially at first, but most everybody who starts an exercise program and sticks with it, begins to see results. Seeing results is great encouragement to stick with it. The benefit you obtain and gains you experience are worth the pains you feel.

In John 5, Jesus asks an invalid man, "Do you want to be well?" The man explains that he previously has tried to get well by entering a pool (or at least he was trying to get some comfort from his distress) but he was prevented by his disabilities. At first you might think that this man was making an excuse. What he was really saying is "Yes. I'd like to be well, but I have things preventing me from achieving that goal." Scripture records what happens next, "Then Jesus said to him, 'Get up! Pick up your mat and walk.' At once the man was cured; he picked up his mat and walked" (John 5:8-9).

Are you giving excuses or do you have a legitimate reason for your inactivity? Are you telling God and others that you want to be well? Are you telling Him and others that you truly want to improve your condition? Or are you just sitting on your mat? Jesus stands at the door to command you to "Get up off your couch and walk." Will you obey?

Lie #3: I don't have access to exercise or health programs/ clubs?

While health clubs and exercise facilities are quite prevalent today, they are not everywhere. Small towns sometimes don't have them and larger cities may have them, but are too far away without access to transportation. As I mentioned above, you don't need access to exercise or health programs and clubs in order to exercise. You can just walk.

A good walking program is found on walkytalk.com. It's a free service by the Blue Cross and Blue Shield Association and it explains in simple, easy-to-understand terms, how and why a free walking program can benefit you. Until mid-2009, this program was endorsed and practiced by Ernie Harwell, a then 91-year-old Christian believer and former broadcaster for the Detroit Tigers Major League Baseball team. Ernie has been struggling from inoperable cancer, but he has led an active, long life and walking helped him achieve it.

If you have the means, you can also do things like install a basketball hoop in your driveway, walk to the nearest lake, ocean or river to take a swim, or do calisthenics or floor routines like sit-ups, push-ups and pull ups in your own home. Get creative. Get to exercising. And stick with it.

Lie #4: Health clubs and programs are too expensive.

Health clubs can cost from $30 a month on up. In today's cost-conscious world, that money can often be spent on other essentials like food and rent. But, if you spend money on luxury items, like cable TV, subscriptions, and other discretionary-income items, you can afford a health club. Look at your budget and see if you really need that $150 a month premium cable TV service that you rarely watch anyway.

I'll also remind you of the advice I gave above in response to Lie #3. You don't have to spend money to exercise. God gave you two legs. Use them! If your neighborhood isn't safe to walk around, take your car, bus or train to a location that is safe. Save the money you would spend on snacks for a year and then go buy a treadmill, and walk inside your own home.

My Exercise Journey

I believe an essential reason why I'm feeling great at 88 is that I regularly, faithfully exercise. There are people 10, 20 or more years younger than myself, who have let their bodies go. They haven't exercised, and as a result, they are not enjoying great health like I am. I think you could and should have great health, too, and an essential ingredient to that health is exercise.

As far back as I can remember I have been a competitor. My dad and mom were competitors and we enjoyed playing competitive games as a family. We played lots of card and table games, but we also played active, recreational games. Sometimes we improvised games like throwing washers into little holes in the dirt in the yard, but we also played more active, organized games, too. We played Ping Pong (or Table Tennis), soccer, softball, football, basketball, and baseball. When I was four, my father taught me tennis. I really enjoy and seem to thrive on competition, and this has translated into being more active. Competition compels me to push my body harder, faster, and longer. I've also found I had to learn to be a good loser before I could become a consistent and a good winner.

Today, I continue to compete and get plenty of exercise. Daily I do floor exercises, plus calisthenics standing up. I walk a mile or so each morning, and I belong to the Soule Park Senior Men's Golf Club. You must be 55 or over to join, and we have around 100 members. We play a different tournament each week, usually on Mondays. We pay annual dues, plus tournament fees, plus green and cart fees. Winners get credit in the Pro Shop for food, merchandise, and cart fees. It is great competition and fellowship. In addition to all the walking I do on the golf course, I do a lot of running when I play tennis every week. I've never belonged to a health club because I believe it is an unnecessary expense. Why not experience the joy of competitive sports yourself? Who knows? Perhaps we'll someday meet out on a golf course or tennis court!

Biblical Ideas on Strength

The physical and spiritual layers of health heavily rely on each other when we look at the word "strength" and how it is used in the Bible. Your spiritual health and your physical health are greatly interconnected, and it is God who gives you strength. The word "strong" is listed in the Bible 231 times, and the word "strength," "strengthen" or "strengthened" is listed 237 times. Bible verses like, "The LORD is my strength and my song; He has become my salvation. He is my God, and I will praise Him, my father's God, and I will exalt Him," epitomize the reoccurring theme that the God of the Bible is the energy and force that empowers mankind. Furthermore, the God of the Bible wants everyone to recognize and acknowledge that *He* is the source of that energy and force.

When people shun God or forget that He is the source of their power and strength, then their health suffers. Let's look again at the story of the Israelites in the desert. God had delivered them from the Egyptians in dramatic fashion (after plagues, the parting of the Red Sea, etc.) and God had provided them with free food in the desert (manna and quail). He also led them in dramatic fashion to the Promised Land, with a pillar of fire by night and a pillar of cloud by day

(Exod. 13:22). They had everything they needed and God was showing up, time and time again, in a big way.

There was no way the Israelites could ignore God – and yet they did. They made a golden calf and worshipped that false god instead. God wasn't amused. Exodus 32: 9-10 reports, "I have seen these people," the LORD said to Moses, "and they are a stiff necked people. Now leave Me alone so that My anger may burn against them." Moses, intervenes, and said, "Oh, LORD, why should Your anger burn against Your people, whom You brought out of Egypt with great power and a mighty hand? Why should the Egyptians say, 'It was with evil intent that He brought them out, to kill them in the mountains and to wipe them off the face of the earth. Turn from Your fierce anger; relent and do not bring disaster on Your people'" (Exod. 32:11-12).

What does God do? First, he makes the Israelites drink a nasty concoction made out of water and ashes from the burnt gold idol. Then, He asks the Israelites through Moses "Who is for Me?" The Levites, a tribe of the Israelites, step forward. Then, in an event that would strike the fear of the LORD into almost anyone, God commands the Levites to kill those who rejected God. "About three thousand of the people died." (Exod. 32:28)

Today, God apparently does not command such drastic measures, but the consequence of rejecting God are still the same: poor health and death. Obedience and recognition of the God of the Bible as your source of strength and power are still required. "For the LORD your God is a consuming fire, a jealous God." (Deut. 4:24)

Hence, it is always good to remember these words, "For

in Him we live and move and have our being." As some of your own poets have said, "We are His offspring" (Acts 17:28). When we recognize that God is our strength, we position ourselves to receive His blessing, and not His wrath or punishment. In and through Him, we stand a greater chance of great health.

In Conclusion

God loves you very much and He wants to have a relationship with you. He wants to give you an abundant life. And, life on this earth can be abundant, filled with a variety of enjoyable activities. One of God's first activities with man was fellowshipping with him in the Garden of Eden. God wants to fellowship with you, too, in your home, at work, at play, and while you exercise. He wants to show you His love by helping you improve your body through exercise. He also wants to use you and your body to bless others, such as your family, your friends, your church, and those who need to hear the Gospel and be discipled to. You are a relational being, created for a purpose.

To improve our life, God has given us two kinds of exercise: Aerobic and Anaerobic. Aerobic exercise involves or improves oxygen consumption by the body. It strengthens the heart and builds endurance. Anaerobic exercise triggers anaerobic metabolism and helps improve strength, speed and power. This is the exercise that improves muscle mass. Both types of exercise are essential for great health. And both kinds can be practiced well into your senior years. You may need to adjust or adapt your program due to your limitations; check with your doctor before starting any exercise program, but exercise will help keep you limber, sharp and strong to function well and serve God as long as He gives you breath.

I think the best exercise is done outdoors. Getting outside is essential for people of all ages, but especially children, because outside is where you get free Vitamin D – from the sun! Vitamin D prevents us from getting debilitating diseases like rickets and other bone softening diseases. When you exercise outdoors, not only do you help your heart, circulatory system, and muscles, but you also help your bones! As you exercise and praise God for giving you life and strength, you'll improve your body and hopefully, have some fun doing it.

In the next section, ***Layer Three: Emotional Health***, I'll examine how and why great spiritual and physical health contributes to great emotional health. I'll explore emotions, conflict, stress, peace, contentment, and Godly relationships. You'll discover how God blesses you with good emotions as a tool for enjoying life and more effective usefulness for His purposes.

Footnotes

1. http://www.time.com/time/health/article/0,8599,1692184,00.html?iid=sphere-inline-sidebar.

Layer Three: Emotional Health

Chapter 8
Handling Conflict and Stress

Peace I leave with you; My peace I give you. I do not give to you as the world gives. Do not let your hearts be troubled and do not be afraid.
- John 14:27

He [Jesus] got up and rebuked the wind and the raging waters; the storm subsided, and all was calm. - Luke 8:25

In 1963, when I was 41 years old, I entered Dr. Van Pelt's office in Tulsa, OK with a problem. I thought my gall bladder was mal-functioning and I felt like it needed to be removed. Pain was my daily companion. My every move, including work and home life, was overshadowed by what felt like a large thorn in my belly. I fully expected the doctor to comply with my request and book the surgery, but he looked me straight in the face and told me, "Dick. There's nothing worse in this world than self-pity." This is not what I expected to hear. I wanted my problem to be purely physical, but he was saying I created my own physical problem by feeling sorry for myself. Ultimately, I was greatly relieved I didn't have to go through with surgery.

My next step was to see a clinical psychologist. He told

me, "You don't like to take responsibility, right?" It was hard to admit, but I agreed with him. "Yes," I said, "you are right. I do avoid responsibility." I decided then and there to own up to my self-pity and avoidance of responsibility. Those two sins were creating emotional and physical stress in me that I could no longer ignore. I, therefore, repented of my sin, and began to pursue God's answers over these issues. Remarkably, my gall bladder also began to feel better.

During this time, I discovered that I created my own physical problems by letting myself be overtaken by fear of responsibility, and worry over uncontrollable outcomes in my life. Since I felt little or no control over my circumstances, I began to feel sorry for myself and sank into self-pity. Stress was eating me from the inside out, taking away my great health. Yet, as I released my worries and fears to God, and accepted responsibility for my thoughts and actions, my health began to improve. I realized I had not completely surrendered all of my life to the Lordship of Jesus Christ, nor had I completely sought the guidance of the Holy Spirit. When I submitted myself to more of God's leadership, and hence, took personal responsibility for the things in my life I had previously avoided, God improved my physical, mental, emotional and spiritual health.

You may have a great life and a great job with lots of responsibility and fun challenges, or you may have a difficult life and no job at all, and feel the weight of life crashing down around you. But if your lifestyle is killing you and causing you undue stress, then you need to seek the God of the Bible and find out how He would want you to live.

Why Worry? Why Fear?

Do you live a life of self-pity, worry, and irresponsibility like I did? Do you let the stresses and cares of life (and/or the consequences of avoiding responsibility) rob you of great emotional strength and health? Do you feel like you don't have enough peace in your life? Is your ability to serve and praise God compromised by runaway emotions? While there is no quick fix to some emotional troubles (professional counseling may be required), the Bible has a lot to say about worry and stress. There is Someone who can unburden you and fill you with the strength and power you need to live a life of victory and not defeat. That person is the God of the Bible.

1 Peter 5:6-7 says, "Humble yourselves, therefore, under God's mighty hand, that He may lift you up in due time. Cast all your anxiety on Him because He cares for you." He invites us to approach Him with humility, recognizing that He is the solution to our problems, and in due time, He will lift us up. It may not be in the timing you want, but He is always there, always faithful, always pulling for you.

Also remember this: His ways are not our ways. His thoughts are not our thoughts. He may take His time or answer you in a way that you don't expect, in order to show you His sovereignty. God is not a vending machine. You don't just order your requests to Him and expect great health in return. It doesn't work like that. (Compare it to a child who only talks to his or her father with his or her own demands. If you were his or her father, you'd be upset about that.) The God of the Bible wants a relationship with you. He wants your heart and He wants a dynamic relationship with you. As you learn to sit at His feet and hear from Him, you can learn how to live optimally, full of increasing opportunities for greater health. (See ***Chapter 16: How to Begin to Enjoy***

Great Eternal Health.)

We shouldn't merely give mental assent that God is there and can help us. We must enter His presence with humbleness, and ask Him to take our burdens. Tell Him your likes and dislikes. Tell Him your heart. And, ask Him for His solutions. Ask the Holy Spirit to lead and guide you in paths of righteousness for His namesake. This means asking Him to show you the right way to go. Then wait on Him, and/or study His word to find an answer.

Do you recognize these hymn lyrics? "When peace like a river, attendeth my way, When sorrows like sea billows roll; Whatever my lot, Thou hast taught me to say, It is well, it is well, with my soul." These are the opening words of the well known hymn by Horatio Spafford, "It is Well with my Soul." Spafford wrote this hymn after a series of traumatic events in his life. First, his son died unexpectedly. Then the Great Chicago Fire left him ruined financially. Then, four daughters drowned while en route to Europe after their ship was struck by another boat and sank. Spafford's wife survived and after she arrived in Europe, she sent him this chilling telegram, "Saved Alone." Despite these series of horrors (that would make many people want to curse God and live a life of bitterness), Spafford humbled himself before God, and learned how to hear and receive from God the healing words that allowed him to say, "It is well with my soul."

Trust in God

Jesus knows this world is sin-wracked and difficult to endure. In John 16:33, Jesus told His followers, "I have told you these things, so that in Me you may have peace. In this world you will have trouble. But take heart! I have overcome the world." What fantastic news this is! We don't have to fight all the junk that comes into our lives. God saves us from sin and the effects of sin, and the stresses of life that weigh us down. He is our shield and guardian.

One way to gain Christ's victory in your life is to completely trust in God and sign your life over to His care. Let's analyze the Bible story about the three Hebrew children: Shadrach, Meshach and Abednego. They defied their unrighteous king and chose to follow the One True God instead. The text is found in Daniel 3:14-22. "King Nebuchadnezzar said to them, 'Is it true, Shadrach, Meshach and Abednego, that you do not serve my gods or worship the image of gold I have set up?'" (Here the leading, popular authority, King Nebuchadnezzar, was questioning and scolding the Israelites for not worshiping the current god of the day. Today, so-called authorities like pop culture icons and our own government often discourage us and try to penalize us for following the God of the Bible.)

Nebuchadnezzar continues, "Now when you hear the sound of the horn, flute, zither, lyre, harp, pipes and all kinds of music, if you are ready to fall down and worship the image I made, very good. But if you do not worship it, you will be thrown immediately into a blazing furnace. Then what god will be able to rescue you from my hand?" (The King thinks he has the upper-hand here when he threatens death. Sometimes our lives are threatened too, and the end seems near, but this is when the God of the Bible is able to show up and show His power.)

"Shadrach, Meshach and Abednego replied to the king, 'O Nebuchadnezzar, we do not need to defend ourselves before you in this matter. If we are thrown into the blazing furnace, the God we serve is able to save us from it, and He will rescue us from your hand, O king.'" (This is where their faith is truly put to the test. They were found to completely rely on God.)

They said, "But even if He does not, we want you to know, O king, that we will not serve your gods or worship the image of gold you have set up." (The Hebrews had pre-determined to follow God, no matter the cost.)

"Then Nebuchadnezzar was furious with Shadrach, Meshach and Abednego, and his attitude toward them changed. He ordered the furnace heated seven times hotter than usual and commanded some of the strongest soldiers in his army to tie up Shadrach, Meshach and Abednego and throw them into the blazing furnace. So these men, wearing their robes, trousers, turbans and other clothes, were bound and thrown into the blazing furnace. The king's command was so urgent and the furnace so hot that the flames of the fire killed the soldiers who took up Shadrach, Meshach and Abednego, and these three men, firmly tied, fell into the blazing furnace. Then King Nebuchadnezzar leaped to his feet in amazement and asked his advisers, 'Weren't there three men that we tied up and threw into the fire?' They replied, 'Certainly, O king.' He said, 'Look! I see four men walking around in the fire, unbound and unharmed, and the fourth looks like a son of the gods.'"

That fourth man in the fire was an angel, sent by God to protect Shadrach, Meshach and Abednego. When they came out of the furnace, they were not burned and their robes did not even smell like smoke. Their faithfulness to God, their willingness to face adversity, and their triumph over adversity earned them a special place in Nebuchadnezzar's administration. They were promoted for their faithfulness.

Now, you may never face anything as scary or adverse as the threat of being thrown into a fire, and my heart goes out to those who are slain by unrighteous governments, but faithfulness to the God of the Bible has its rewards. If you are killed by an unrighteous ruler because of your faith, you'll spend a wonderful eternity with your Lord. If you are spared by God because of your faithfulness, you might even be promoted or given an earthly blessing. Either way, it's a win-win situation. Faithfulness has its privileges.

Give Thanks Always

King David, of the Old Testament, got it right when he wrote, "I will extol the LORD at all times; His praise will always be on my lips" (Ps. 34:1). If you can get into a habit of continual praise (like David did), your spirit will remain high because it is difficult to be in a bad mood when you are counting your blessings. By willfully acknowledging the goodness and gifts of God, you force your mind and spirit to be positive.

The Apostle Paul, in the New Testament, echoes these words, "Rejoice in the Lord always. I will say it again: Rejoice!" (Eph. 4:4). In this world you'll face many troubles. You could respond with a life full of complaints. Or you could praise God anyway. Life is too short to focus on your pains. If you are praising God or giving Him thanks, then you aren't grumbling or complaining.

"Rejoicing always" may seem like a bit of pop-psychology, but it works and it's Biblical. It's the same as looking at the glass half-full, rather than half-empty. If your mind and heart are fixed on Christ and His goodness, then you are focusing on what you have rather than on what you don't have, on the positive rather than the negative. A very popular song of yesteryear stressed this important truth with lyrics about "accentuating the positive, eliminating the negative, latching onto the affirmative, and not messing with

Mr. In-Between." [1] Fear and worry will tell you to look away from Christ, but the following command is better. "Taste and see that the LORD is good; blessed is the man who takes refuge in Him." (Ps. 34:8)

Allow me to list a few scriptures of God's goodness and grace, encouraging you to recognize how marvelous and awesome He really is:

- "The heavens declare the glory of God; the skies proclaim the work of His hands." (Ps. 19:1)

- "And my God will meet *all* your needs according to His glorious riches in Christ Jesus." (Phil. 4:19)

- "Jesus did many other things as well. If every one of them were written down, I suppose that even the whole world would not have room for the books that would be written." (John 21:25).

- "Give thanks to the LORD, for He is good; His love endures forever." (1 Chron. 16:34)

If you have been a Christian believer for a long time but God seems far away, then these scriptures may not significantly rally you enough to move into thanks and praise. If your faith seems dry, ask God for a fresh anointing of His Holy Spirit. As the Psalmist writes in 51:12, "Restore to me the joy of Your Salvation and grant me a willing spirit, to sustain me." Even if times are tough for you, God wants you filled with praise, power and His glory. From the Hebrew children thrown into the fiery furnace, to David in front of Goliath, to Jonah in the Belly of the whale, and Job hit with calamity after calamity,

God demonstrates His faithfulness to role models of faith throughout Scripture. These are ordinary men and women, who endure under the most vile, awful conditions, and yet are able to retain their faith, peace and joy. It's not impossible.

1 Thessalonians 5:18 says, "Give thanks in all circumstances, for this is God's will for you in Christ Jesus." If your car breaks down, thank and praise the Lord. If your marriage is suffering, thank and praise the Lord for your spouse. If your house needs repairs, your children are running wild, or if you're having trouble at work, thank and praise the Lord. You might say, "But Dick, you don't know my spouse." Or "You don't know my boss. He (or She) is so awful." Your spouse, boss, children or person offending you may be filled with the Devil himself, but God says, "Praise Me. Trust Me. Don't complain. Don't worry."

If we cast all our cares on God, trust Him with the outcome, give thanks in all things, and ask the Holy Spirit to guide you and lead you into all truth, then you stand a much better chance at great emotional (and physical) health than if you resort to anger, complaining and worry. (It's important to recognize the difference here between difficulty and abuse. If you are being abused by another, seek God for safety and look for opportunities to escape. I'm just trying to tell you that God is able to redeem and restore even in the most difficult of circumstances.)

Read these words from 1 Peter 5:8-11. "Be self-controlled and alert. Your enemy the devil prowls around like a roaring lion looking for someone to devour. Resist him, standing firm in the faith, because you know that your brothers throughout the world are undergoing the same kind of sufferings. And the God of all grace, Who called you to His eternal glory in Christ, after you have suffered a little while, will Himself restore you and make you strong, firm and steadfast. To Him be the power for ever and ever. Amen." What a great and precious promise! God, Himself, will restore you.

Take comfort in the final words that Jesus shared with His disciples before He descended into heaven. For the last three years prior to this moment, Jesus lived with His disciples. He ate with them, drank with them, walked with them, and lived life with them. They were completely dependent on Him and they had come to rely on His presence. But, Jesus knew He was about to leave them. He knew He would not again appear to them as a man in bodily form. So Jesus gave them these words of encouragement, which are meant for all disciples, even today.

"But the Counselor, the Holy Spirit, whom the Father will send in My name, will teach you all things and will remind you of everything I have said to you. Peace I leave with you; My peace I give you. I do not give to you as the world gives. Do not let your hearts be troubled and do not be afraid." (John 14:26-28)

In Him, we have supernatural peace. Not peace based on circumstance or good fortune, but by the presence and fellowship of the Holy Spirit. These are exciting words, that disciples of Christ can still embrace.

Untouchable Stress

The word stress has many meanings, but the definition relating to a person's health is "physical, mental, or emotional strain or tension." More specifically, it's "a specific response by the body to a stimulus, as fear or pain that disturbs or interferes with the normal physiological equilibrium of an organism."[2]

Stress is an unavoidable part of life. Even before sin came into this world through Adam and Eve's error, mankind had tasks to do on this earth. He had to get up and go to work, taking care of the garden. He had challenges to face and problems to solve by his own effort. The garden was perfect, but it needed minding and tending. Part of the joy and fun of life is problem-solving and using your God-given mind and body to tackle the challenges of life. Stress is only a bad word if it becomes unmanageable.

I deal with stress every day of my life. Most of the time, I can manage it. But sometimes, I don't know how to handle it and that is when I must fall on my face in humility and gain strength and guidance from my Holy God. I honestly believe that if I didn't have my Christian faith, then this daily stress would have put me in the grave. Without God, I would have succumbed to the stresses of this world, developed health problems, and possibly died. I give 100% credit to God's Holy Spirit for daily advising me on how to successfully handle stress so that it doesn't touch my health adversely.

I honestly and sincerely say, "Praise God for stress." Be it mental, physical, emotional, spiritual, moral, economic, marital or whatever. Again I say, "Praise God!" The reason I praise God for stress is that I believe that, "All things work together for good for those who love God and are called according to His purposes" (Rom 8:28). Whether stress is a result of my own error, someone else's behavior, uncontrollable events from God's original design or Satan's plan, I respond as the Apostle James wrote in James 1:2-5. "Consider it pure joy, my brothers, whenever you face trials of many kinds, because you know that the testing of your faith develops perseverance. Perseverance must finish its work so that you may be mature and complete, not lacking anything. If any of you lacks wisdom, he should ask God, who gives generously to all without finding fault, and it will be given to him."

I ask God for wisdom and I persevere. I realize this is a mature stance and a potentially difficult challenge to meet. But, those who stand up to the stress of the world with praise, thanks and joy on their lips (and those who appeal to God for Wisdom) will reap a great reward of peace, whatever the events that transpire. If you develop this attitude and stance, then nothing can touch you.

Read these words from Psalm 46:1-2: "God is our refuge and strength, an ever-present help in trouble. Therefore we will not fear, though the earth give way and the mountains fall into the heart of the sea, though its waters roar and foam and the mountains quake with their surging." Those are some dramatic words, and great promises. They are armor for those who read and believe it, to stand up to and endure the world's most deadly stresses. Those words are a great source of comfort and strength to me and I hope they become your source of strength and comfort too.

Footnotes

1. http://en.wikipedia.org/wiki/Accentuate_The_Positive.
2. http://dictionary.reference.com/browse/stress.

Chapter 9
Right Relationships

And so we know and rely on the love God has for us. God is love. Whoever lives in love lives in God, and God in him. - 1 John 4:16

On one occasion an expert in the law stood up to test Jesus. "Teacher," he asked, "what must I do to inherit eternal life?" "What is written in the Law?" he replied. "How do you read it?" He answered: "Love the Lord your God with all your heart and with all your soul and with all your strength and with all your mind; and, Love your neighbor as yourself." "You have answered correctly," Jesus replied. "Do this and you will live."
- Luke 10:25-28

The God of the Bible insists on being #1 in the lives of His followers. Anytime we put anyone or anything ahead of God the Father, Son and Holy Spirit, we are in error. We are making an idol for ourselves, and worshipping a false god. We are minimizing and disrespecting the One True God. The result we experience is dysfunctional, bad relationships top to bottom. We are out of sorts with God and man.

In my first marriage, I allowed my feelings for my wife to supersede my feelings for the God of the Bible. I thought this was what marriages were supposed to be. After all, the Bible says, "Husband, love your wives" (Eph. 5:25). I took this to include giving away to her my God-given authority to be head of the home. I thought I was doing a loving, respectful act by letting her take responsibility for major decisions in the home. I was wrong. I neglected being the man that God wanted me and expected me to be. As such, I was in sin. I needed to repent and change.

My first wife often tried to make me change. She tried to make me see the error of my ways, but I was hard-headed and never got the message. I thought she wasn't appreciating the great love I was trying to give her, by letting her rule the household. Surely, she must respect the fact that I was trying to make her a "liberated" woman. Despite my efforts, I was creating a negative effect in our relationship. Our family suffered greatly. I now chalk up my foolishness to immaturity and lack of understanding.

My first marriage ended in divorce. When I married my second wife, Margaret Ann, I unfortunately fell into the same pattern. I became afraid of controversial topics with her. I avoided making difficult decisions. I wanted peace at any price. I feared to take a stand on what I believed was best for our marriage and family. I feared I'd lose the love and approval of my wife, if I took a stand. I didn't want to pay the price of leadership, but by not paying the price, I hurt both of us. She desperately needed me to take the reins, but I wasn't doing it.

Despite my sin and error, I felt *completely* responsible for her happiness and well-being. I wanted our marriage to succeed, but I just did not know how. Or if I did, I was not moving in the direction that would make our marriage succeed for fear that it would rock the boat. In the early 2000s, the Holy Spirit convicted me of my sin. God showed me that I identified myself with being a little boy. I realized I needed to "grow up" and become the man God expected me to be. Convicted of my error, I repented of my sins immediately. Almost overnight, I began to stick to what I believed to be true and right for our marriage. I held to my convictions, even if it meant temporary discord in the home. Yet, the more I led, the more I realized that I was previously acting like a coward. I was just like a little boy who gave-in to his parents. So, for several years now, I have been thinking and behaving more and more like a real man. The consequences of these decisions have held radical results.

Amazingly, both Margaret Ann and I have experienced a dramatic decrease in our conflict and stress. She doesn't feel the weight of responsibility for major decisions in our home, and hence, she is happier. She feels glad that she isn't taking away my God-given right to lead the home. She's glad she isn't contributing to my improper state of immaturity and boyishness. All around, she's a much happier person, and so am I. We have both matured, and grown in the Lord. We disagree a lot less than before.

She has become an even more wonderful wife, an even better companion and co-worker with me in ministry. I give her tremendous credit in helping me get to where I am today. Her love for God, and her love, respect, appreciation and support for me has enabled me to realize my shortcomings and to strive for my potential. She gave me the freedom and the space I needed to be able to repent and make the God of the Bible #1 in my life. I've come to realize that when I put God #1 in my life and give Him more love and respect (through obedience and faith in Him) than the love and respect I give to my other relationships, (including the relationship with my wife), then all my relationships fall in line. I serve other people best by serving God, first and foremost. My wife, family and friends are the beneficiaries of my love for God because they relate to a man of God, who is living and loving correctly.

Let Love Rule

I truly believe the key to every good relationship is to love God first and foremost and *then* love your neighbor as yourself. (These are the great commandments given by Jesus in Matthew 26:36-39.) If we can't love ourselves, it would be difficult or impossible to love others. When you keep these priorities of love in order, then *all* your relationships function optimally. Think about this. If everyone followed these commands and let the law of love rule over their lives, then problems in the world would be greatly diminished. I'm not talking about some kind of pie-in-the-sky, hippie utopia here. I'm talking about living in this world of sin and decay, but responding to others just as God would respond to them – following God's marching orders to love Him, first, and others as ourselves. Most (but not all) of our problems would vanish because Satan is still loose, wrecking havoc wherever he can. But if God were loved and obeyed first and foremost instead of money, power, greed, and selfishness, then the world would be a much better, different, and healthier place.

What is love anyway? First, let's find out what it is not. 1 Corinthians 13:1-3 tells us the answer. "If I speak in the tongues of men and of angels, but have not love, I am only a resounding gong or a clanging cymbal. If I have the gift of prophecy and can fathom all mysteries and all knowledge, and if I have a faith that can move mountains, but have not love, I am nothing. If I give all I possess to the poor and surrender my body to the flames, but have not love, I gain nothing." In other words, love isn't about showy religious performance. Do not confuse great works done in the name of "ministry" with loving others. Creating programs, speaking eloquently, and building a church that draws thousands does not equal love. When all the "religious acts" are done for the day, are you acting in love towards others? Jesus came to live a sacrificial life of service to humanity. He came to meet their physical, spiritual, emotional and mental needs by demonstrating practical love. He ate, shared, lived with and shared life with others. So should you.

So again, the question is raised. What is love? A continuation of 1 Corinthians 13 in verses 4-8 tell us plainly. "Love is patient, love is kind. It does not envy, it does not boast, it is not proud. It is not rude, it is not self-seeking, it is not easily angered, it keeps no record of wrongs. Love does not delight in evil but rejoices with the truth. It always protects, always trusts, always hopes, always perseveres. Love never fails." These brief words contain the secret to success for every human relationship.

The Apostle Paul wrote these words to the Corinthians, because they, like we, forgot what it meant to act in love.

With the pressures of the world bearing down, it's easy to act unloving. We first see these words demonstrated to us by the God of the Bible. Time and time again through the Old Testament and also through the person and presence of Jesus Christ, we see God acting out these attributes of love to all mankind. We are able to access this God-type love through asking the Holy Spirit to live in us, guiding us into all Truth, and empowering us to live as Christ did.

1 John 4:19-20 sums up the matter on love. "We love because He first loved us. If anyone says, 'I love God,' yet hates his brother, he is a liar. For anyone who does not love his brother, whom he has seen, cannot love God, whom he has not seen." We are able to love others because God first loved us. We respond to God with love, because we know, feel and experience His redemptive, atoning love for us. With that tangible profound love lavished upon us, it is much easier to give love to our fellow men.

What happens if we don't *feel* loved by God? How can we respond in love to Him or share love with others? These are times when we must act in mere obedience, even when we don't *feel* like it. You don't have to *feel* love in order to act in love. Do you think Jesus felt like dying on the cross? Hebrews 12:2 says Jesus "who for the joy set before Him endured the cross." Jesus obeyed and experienced a very painful death, to experience the joy of redeeming mankind. Sometimes love demands delayed gratification.

So again, when God commands us to "Love one another as I have loved you, so you must love one another" (John 13:34), it sometimes is an act of the will. And when God says, "Be devoted to one another in brotherly love. Honor one another above yourselves" (Rom. 12:10), it sometimes requires a deliberate choice. It might be difficult to love an unlovable person, but when we act in obedience, God will be glorified and righteousness will be fulfilled. There is no excuse not to love. God commands it. The Holy Spirit in you can make it happen. Love is a verb that must be expressed in action in order to be fulfilled.

The Types of Love

The Greeks have four definitions for the word "Love." Let's look at these definitions and see how we can apply them to our lives, in order to improve our own health and the health of those lives we touch.

These four Greek words for love are Agape (a noun with the verb agapao), Philo, Eros, and Storge. Briefly said, Agape is divine love; Philo is friendship love; Eros is sensual or physical love; and Storge is familial love. Note philo is the same root word used in the larger word philosophy, meaning love of wisdom. Eros is used derivatively in erotic. All four loves have played and continue to play important roles in my health.

It is interesting to read that Jesus uses agape in John 15:15-17, "I no longer call you servants, because a servant does not know his master's business. Instead, I have called you friends, for everything that I learned from My Father I have made known to you. You did not choose Me, but I chose you and appointed you to go and bear fruit—fruit that will last. Then the Father will give you whatever you ask in My name. This is My command: *Love* each other." Jesus is asking His disciples to love as God loves, sacrificially, without regard to whether or not the recipient gives love in return. This is as C.S. Lewis states, "The Greatest Love."[1]

Look at this passage from John 21:15-17: "Jesus said to Simon Peter, 'Simon, son of John, do you truly *love* Me more than these?' 'Yes, Lord,' he said, 'You know that I *love* You.' Jesus said, 'Feed My lambs.' Again Jesus said, 'Simon son of John, do you truly *love* Me?' He answered, 'Yes, Lord, You know that I *love* You.' Jesus said, 'Take care of My sheep.' The third time He said to him, 'Simon son of John, do you *love* Me?' Peter was hurt because Jesus asked him the third time, 'Do you *love* Me?' He said, 'Lord, You know all things; You know that I *love* You.' Jesus said, 'Feed My sheep.'"

At first glance, this passage seems to be about Peter getting his feelings hurt when Jesus asks him the same question repeatedly. What is actually being said here is deeper and cannot be fully appreciated because we are limited with our English understanding of the word "love." Remember, the Greeks have four words for love and the original text makes a distinction between the different meanings and usage of the word "love."

The first two times Jesus addresses Peter, he uses the word Agapao. He is asking, "Peter, do you love Me with a divine love." Peter, unable to commit to this type of love, replies "Yes Lord. You know I Philo You." Peter was saying, "I love You with a friendship love." Philo suggests a love over a common activity or interest. They were both happy together doing ministry, but Peter felt Jesus was pushing him a little too far. When Jesus addresses Peter a third time, "Simon, son of Peter, do you love Me," Jesus goes down to Peter's level and uses the Philo word for love. I think Peter was sad that Jesus was not only questioning his love for Him, but Peter was also feeling sad for himself that he couldn't love as Jesus asked him to love. Do you love Jesus with a divine love or a friendship love? If you do not love God with all your heart, mind, soul and body, then ask God to fill you with the Holy Spirit to love as God loves.

Romans 12:10 is an example of storge love. "Be devoted to one another in brotherly love. Honor one another above yourselves." This is a love that is familiar, and often easy to practice. It's the natural love that family members feel for one another. But since Paul made a point of commanding it to Christ's disciples, it must have been an issue for early Christians. This inter-connected type of love between the members of the body of Christ is essential in order for the works and goals of Christ to be fully accomplished through the Church. After all, the love the Church holds for one-another is a testament to the truth of our belief and the uniqueness of our faith.

Eros Misapplied

The Greek word Eros does not appear in the biblical text, but the Biblical text is quite clear on how sexual love is to be practiced and applied. The only appropriate context for sexual love is between a man and woman, who are married to each other. Their shared love through expressions of intimacy is not only God's original plan for married heterosexual couples, but it is also a beautiful private reflection of Christ's love with His bride, the Church. Homosexuality perverts that plan (and Holy example) and therefore is not Biblically or morally acceptable.

Here are some scriptures on homosexual practices.

- "If a man lies with a man as one lies with a woman, both of them have done what is detestable. They must be put to death; their blood will be on their own heads." (Lev. 20:13)

- "Do you not know that the wicked will not inherit the kingdom of God? Do not be deceived: Neither the sexually immoral nor idolaters nor adulterers nor male prostitutes nor homosexual offenders nor thieves nor the greedy nor drunkards nor slanderers nor swindlers will inherit the kingdom of God." (1 Cor. 6:9-10)

Despite this clear message, homosexuals today, in every State, are pushing for moral and legal equivalency with their behavior. They figure if they are legally and morally protected, then their unnatural acts can be justified. Yet, they fail to realize that the acts reserved for marriage alone are sacred, created by God to reflect the sacred love shared by Christ and His Church. Eros is only to be practiced between a married man and woman. Marriage has existed since the creation of Adam and Eve. And just because modern times and the gay agenda are trying to make homosexual practices and relationships more palatable, the old, old truths of Scriptures remain.

I have come to learn about an Atlanta, Georgia man, whom I'll call Allen. Allen lived the gay lifestyle for 20 years, having many sexual encounters with multiple men. After a lover left him, Allen cried out to God, and God replied to Allen saying, "The homosexual lifestyle is not what I intended for you. Come out." This Word (which is in agreement with Scripture) put the Fear of God into Allen. This man repented of his sinful behavior, and sought the Lord's forgiveness. Allen lived for a period of time as a celibate man, despite his occasional temptations to act out sexually with other men. Even so, Allen resisted his urges and surrendered his life and sexuality over to God. A few years later, God put a woman, whom I'll call Priscilla (a former lesbian) into Allen's life. They met and developed a kindred spirit with each other. Now, they are in love with each other and are married. They live life as an example to others of what God can do to redeem even the most fractured of lives.

A final notable part of this true story is that Allen still occasionally has temptations to act out sexually towards men. But Allen has made a covenant with God and his wife to not do that. Allen isn't necessarily "cured" of his homosexuality (although God certainly can do that), but Allen has chosen to obey God and live a life of faithfulness to his wife, a gift the Lord has given him. Daily, Allen and his wife learn what it is to die to self, pick up their crosses, and live for Christ. Allen says life isn't necessarily easier living the straight life, but life is definitely better, richer, and healthier. Obedience to God has its rewards.

Sympathy vs. Empathy

As a former pastor, living life and loving God and others as myself, I've found myself in the position of having to offer a lot of sympathy to those in need. Despite my good intentions, I came to realize that I was not faithfully serving my parishioners when I offered them sympathy. Instead of offering sympathy, I should have offered empathy. I came to learn that empathy was more in line with God's Will and much better in the short and long-term for the health of the person I was serving, plus my own health.

Sympathy is the fact or power of sharing the feelings

of another, especially in sorrow or trouble; fellow feeling, compassion, or commiseration.[2] Empathy, on the other hand, is the intellectual identification with or vicarious experiencing of the feelings, thoughts, or attitudes of another.[3] With sympathy, the person you are counseling may take some comfort in that you understand his or her needs, but you are no further in helping them out of their problem. As a sympathizer, all you can do is say, "I understand how you feel," even if you really don't. Empathy, however, goes beyond sympathy and offers a helping hand. It actively searches for identification with the pain being felt by the person in need, but then goes further and objectively offers strength and power to help the person in need out of their troubles.

The best illustration I can think of on the difference between sympathy and empathy is as follows: Two rock climbers are tied to each other for safety reasons, one slips and falls, the other has a choice between sympathy or empathy. Sympathy calls for him to jump after his friend and they both fall to their deaths together. Empathy calls for him to brace himself, keep calm, be ready to hold on when the rope tightens, and then pull his friend to safety.

Christ didn't merely watch humanity from heaven and shake His head saying, "Poor humans." He came down from heaven, lived as one of us, experiencing the same bodily pain and temptations that we do, so that He could completely sympathize and empathize with our experiences. We know Christ can sympathize with us: "For we do not have a high priest who is unable to sympathize with our weaknesses, but we have One who has been tempted in every way, just as we are—yet was without sin" (Heb. 4:15). Yet, Christ also, and more importantly, empathizes with us: "Therefore, He is able to save completely those who come to God through Him, because He always lives to intercede for them." Don't just feel sorry for others. Offer them a helping hand, up and out.

The best way to help another is to appeal to Christ, who is exceedingly able and willing to save.

In Conclusion

In all my 88 years, I have learned a great deal on how to relate biblically with others. Here are some of the greatest lessons I've learned. I've learned how to overcome my tendency from childhood to be a manipulator. I've learned not to be obsessed with life on this earth since it is only the beginning of eternity. And I'm gradually learning not to be an enabler to others to behave in such a way to be contrary to God's Will. I'm learning that a successful and happy Christian marriage cannot be a democracy because God has ordained that the man be the leader of his household. I'm learning to accept God's wrath or anger over sin. If He doesn't tolerate it or accept it, why should I? I'm learning how to express love in all its languages and meanings, every day. I'm learning to accept the thorns in the flesh God has either given me or allowed Satan to inflict on me, so that in perseverance, I can grow as a human. With regards to gifts, I'm learning it is always the thought behind the gift that is important and not the size or monetary value of the gift.

I like to give "strokes" to others and I like to receive "strokes" from others, such as words of affirmation and hugs. Study after study reveals that strokes are important in order to enjoy a full, abundant, and more satisfying life. We need each other, and we need to be supported by each other. This support can be manifested in many ways but it really amounts to being loved, appreciated, encouraged, motivated, forgiven, etc. I believe a big factor in my excellent health is the fact that I have come to seek "strokes" from the God of the Bible, rather than from people. Unfortunately, people often fail me. When this happens, it's easy to feel slighted and feel like my day is ruined. (Life's not fair!)

If I come to rely on my strength and "strokes" from others, I'll end up disappointed and discouraged. When I rely on and receive "strokes" from the God of the Bible, who never fails me, then I am able to give others through Christ the "strokes" they crave. I must admit that I really enjoy and appreciate "strokes" from people in general (and certain ones in particular), but my peace and happiness is not, nor should it be, dependent on what other people do.

In closing, I'd like to look at the words of John 12:42-43: "Yet at the same time many even among the leaders believed in Him (meaning Jesus). But because of the Pharisees, they would not confess their faith for fear they would be put out of the synagogue; for they loved praise from men more than praise from God." When you seek more praise from God than men, you'll gain favor with God and man. You'll be a man (or woman) of God, strong in His might, filled with His power, confident in His love, and operating from a position of purpose.

In the next section ***Layer Four: Mental Health***, I'll talk about how to "think" biblically. I'll talk about ways to keep your mind sharp and ways to think clearly. I'll talk about great financial thoughts, and great political thoughts. I'll explore thinking and responding to the world with a Biblical worldview. When we think "Christianly" about all things, we'll be able to behave and respond in a way that not only pleases God, but will serve and benefit ourselves and those around us.

Footnotes

1. Lewis, C.S., *The Four Loves*; NY:NY, Harcourt; 1991
2. http://dictionary.reference.com/browse/sympathy.
3. http://dictionary.reference.com/browse/Empathy.

Layer Four: Mental Health

Chapter 10
Keeping Your Mind Sharp

For as he thinketh in his heart, so is he.
- Proverbs 23:7 (King James Version)

Finally, brothers, whatever is true, whatever is noble, whatever is right, whatever is pure, whatever is lovely, whatever is admirable—if anything is excellent or praiseworthy—think about such things. - Philippians 4:8

One of the most difficult mental challenges occurred to me in December, 1943 at Notre Dame University. I had enlisted in the U.S. Navy and was thrilled to be selected for Midshipman School (Officers Training). There were close to 200 college students there and most of them had engineering backgrounds and/or were training in the Navy to be civil engineers. Although I was in the Navy, I had no such training. My fellow students seemed to understand the teachings of the Naval engineers going on in the classes, but I was completely lost. I needed help, but I did not know where to find it.

I took the tests but I did not score well. Things went from bad to worse and it became apparent I was flunking out. Suddenly one night, I remembered God's promise in

Philippians 4:13, "I can do everything through Him who gives me strength." I thought I wasn't mentally strong enough to pass the course, but when I saw that verse, read it and claimed it in fervent prayer, I discovered that God was ready to answer my prayer and hold up to His promise.

One of my three roommates, Walter Brunning, was an engineer from Louisville, Kentucky. He had taken a liking to me and asked me if I needed help after I had claimed that promise in prayer. I thought, "Wow. God is good. He does answer prayer." I answered Walter with a definitive "Yes!"

Walter sat down with me and we worked fervently together for several hours. Walter was patient and I was so attentive to his help, that we did not give any thought to the lateness of the hour. We worked past midnight, and around two in the morning, I suddenly experienced clarity in my mind. (I now call it an "Ah-ha moment" or a moment of enlightenment.) It was something I had never experienced before. It was as though I was in a dark room and someone suddenly switched on a light. I turned to Walter and shouted, "I've got it!" All of a sudden, the presentations being made by the Naval engineers made sense to me.

From that moment on, I did extremely well in all my midshipman classes and eventually graduated with honors. I have absolutely no doubt that God sent His Holy Spirit to answer my prayer and He had used my friend, Walter Bruning, to enlighten my mind, heart and soul. Praise God from Whom all blessings flow! (Of course, the Holy Spirit was the one who turned the light on in my mind. Walter was simply the conduit, or channel for bringing God's power to me.) This experience and many others have proven to me without a shadow of a doubt that God not only cares for our souls, spirits, and bodies, but also our minds.

Thinking Vs. Knowing

John 1:1-4 says, "In the beginning was the Word, and the Word was with God, and the Word was God. He was with God in the beginning. Through Him all things were made; without Him nothing was made that has been made. In Him was life, and that life was the light of men. The light shines in the darkness, but the darkness has not understood it."

Using letters and words, which are merely symbols representing real objects and concepts, is a completely cerebral or mental activity. The mind looks at the symbols (words) and makes an association to an actual object or concept. What John is saying in these verses is that God is ultimate reality and one way to understand Him as that ultimate reality is by understanding Him through words or more specifically, His Holy Word. Words describe the God of the Bible, and Words, through audio/visual teaching or through written text, communicate who and what God is. Through His Word (the Holy Scripture), God has revealed Himself to humankind as much as can be expressed and said in the written Word. And to understand this Word, the mind must be completely engaged.

I truly believe a *big factor* in my excellent health is my ability and willingness to *think*, as opposed to *know*. To k*now* is to gather information from one or more of the five senses such as sight, hearing, smell, taste and touch. I know that skies are blue and clouds are white. But I think when the skies turn dark grey that it will probably rain soon. I deduce from facts taken previously, that rain showers, even thunderstorms, follow a darkening of the skies.

Here is another example of deductive reasoning. Notice the third point requires thinking.

1. Tiger Woods is a professional golfer.
2. Professional golfers often appear on television.
3. Tiger Woods often appears on television.

Another form of thinking is inductive reasoning. Here, I take facts to form a theory of a conclusion. The conclusion isn't ensured by the facts, but my facts build a case for the conclusion to be likely true. Here is an example of inductive thinking: If all the ice I have touched in the past is cold, then I believe the ice I will touch in the future will also be cold. Now, there may be ice that exists out there that isn't cold, (and I'd like to know about that type of ice if there is such), but I'm willing to trust that *all* ice is cold because of the observations I have made in the past. Essentially, I'm stepping out in faith, believing a conclusion I can not guarantee, but believe to be true.

I've discovered that as time goes on, more and more people are reluctant to think. They are reluctant to commit themselves to a conclusion based on the evidence they are gathering. Some are afraid they might be wrong. Others simply don't use or haven't used their brains to process information through thinking. If you ask them what they think of such-and-such, they will often reply that they don't know. When I press the issue by saying I only want to know what they *think*, not what they *know*, they often get defensive. Sadly, I think this decline of thinking in our world is evidence of Satan and his demons stealing away from us one of our strongest, most valuable gifts from God: the ability to use our minds.

Skeptics are those who do not commit to a conclusion based on the facts. These kinds of people are today being championed as the wise and learned among us. "Question everything," they say. "Don't jump to conclusions." They hide behind their inconclusiveness, while those who commit to a conclusion are often ridiculed and scoffed at. A perfect example of this is the conclusion that Jesus Christ is God.

Remarkably, a variety of people can look at the same facts about Jesus and can come to different conclusions. The skeptic will look at the facts and claims of Christ's birth, life, death and resurrection, and because the skeptic has a presupposition that Christ is not God, will walk away denying the facts. The skeptic holds onto his old conclusion. The skeptic isn't thinking. He's entrenching himself with lies.

The God of the Bible desires that all men come unto salvation. Yet, if people are stubborn and refuse to believe, then God can and will let them languish in their folly. Look at this verse from Romans 1:28. "Furthermore, since they [Roman homosexuals] did not think it worthwhile to retain the knowledge of God, He [God] gave them over to a depraved mind, to do what ought not to be done." God will never force you to believe or trust in Him, but He will "give you over to a depraved mind" if your heart is set on that. Hence, I do believe there is such a thing as minds that are given over to the enemy (Satan), and unless God performs a supernatural work in the life of the "depraved," they will remain entrenched in their lies.

Can you see how "thinking" and "living by faith" are

closely related? Perhaps they are one and the same. Accepting something by faith requires a great deal of thought. Most of what I do, say, think, and feel is based on what I think is true. That translates into living my life by faith, which is informed by my thinking. And, if I think on the God of the Bible and His Word, then my life will be more in line with the thoughts and life of the Great Teacher, the Holy Spirit. Meditating on God brings a promise. Read these words from Joshua 1:8. "Do not let this Book of the Law depart from your mouth; meditate on it day and night, so that you may be careful to do everything written in it. Then you will be prosperous and successful."

It would be easy to do, say, feel, and think based on group thinking or majority rule. But what if the majority is wrong? I think of lemmings that unknowingly run with the crowd and run off a cliff to their deaths because they are following the majority. Study the claims of Christ. Read challenging books like *Evidence that Demands a Verdict* by Josh McDowell, *Mere Christianity* by C.S. Lewis and *The Case for Christ* by Lee Strobel. Dare to think differently. Dare to think Christ-like. Proverbs 3:13-14 says, "Blessed is the man who finds wisdom, the man who gains understanding, for it is more profitable than silver and yields better returns than gold."

Willing to be Crazy

I applaud and encourage all who would take a step of faith and put their trust in Jesus Christ as their Lord and Savior. Living by faith is not for the faint of heart, but it is a life that Jesus calls *all* His disciples to live. While stepping out in faith to accept Jesus Christ as Lord and Savior requires a leap of faith (as well as some deep thinking), witnessing miracles in our time and finding great, lasting personal growth often requires complete abandonment of the "facts."

The God of the Bible created this world with all its physical laws (or facts). Furthermore, mankind has created a scientific method, which further relies on gathering facts to come to some conclusions. Here is one of God's physical laws: gravity pulls objects earthward. Here is a scientific conclusion by man: except in rare cases after radical surgery, a person crippled from birth will never walk. Faith in Christ can turn these "facts" upside down.

When you become a disciple of Christ, sometimes Christ asks you to abandon the facts, and do some crazy things. One dark and stormy night, when Peter was out fishing, he saw Jesus out walking on the water. (Don't the facts tell us that a man will sink if he tries to walk on water?) Matthew 14:28-29 says, "'Lord, if it's You,' Peter replied, 'tell me to come to You on the water.' 'Come,' He [Jesus] said." Peter got out of the boat, and it wasn't until Peter focused on the wind and waves that he began to sink, to fear and have doubt, but Jesus told Peter to focus on Him, stretched out His hand, and Peter put weight on his feet and the water supported him. Peter walked on water!

Later, after Christ ascended into Heaven (Facts tell us that gravity holds mankind to earth, right?), Peter and John were walking toward the temple to pray. They were interrupted by a crippled man who could not walk from birth. Peter said to him, "In the name of Jesus Christ of Nazareth, walk. Taking him by the right hand, he helped him up, and instantly the man's feet and ankles became strong. He jumped to his feet and began to walk" (Acts 3:6-8).

When you put your faith in the God of the Bible, the God of the Bible can, and sometimes will, do the miraculous. The God of the Bible can supersede the facts and create a new work. In both stories above, Peter took a leap of faith to believe the fact that God loved him and had a purpose for him. Peter believed that "fact" over and above the physical fact that water cannot support the body weight of a man and the medical fact that a man crippled from birth cannot walk.

A final thought on this topic can be found in 1 Corinthians 1:27, "But God chose the foolish things of the world to shame the wise; God chose the weak things of the world to shame the strong." If you are a follower of the God of the Bible, you must believe and be willing to appear foolish before the wise of the world. Believers in the God of the Bible know that God is true to His promises. They accept it as fact. For unbelievers, prayer, belief in miracles or doing something crazy (like walking on water) is foolishness. Are you willing to be a fool for God?

Rationalization

A genuinely dangerous and foolish thing for everyone to do is to rationalize. It's a danger that exists for all who would dare to think. People rationalize when they make something irrational appear rational or reasonable, or they provide a natural explanation of something (as a myth), or they justify one's unacceptable behavior or weaknesses. People who rationalize also find plausible but untrue reasons for their conduct. Those who rationalize think falsely to create temporary favorable conclusions for themselves, or others they are trying to influence.

The first written record we have of rationalization is found in Genesis 3 where Adam blames Eve and Eve blames the serpent. God had told them they could eat freely of all the fruits and vegetables in the Garden of Eden except they were *not* to eat the fruit of the tree of knowledge of good and evil. After the serpent persuaded Eve to eat the forbidden fruit, Eve persuaded Adam to do the same. God eventually confronted Adam with this infraction of the rules and Adam defended his disobedience by blaming Eve, instead of accepting the responsibility himself. God then confronts Eve and she blames the serpent, instead of accepting the responsibility herself. Both Adam and Eve rationalize, which God found unacceptable. God punished them for their disobedience by banishing them from the garden.

Rationalization has been a powerful force in my life as far back as I can remember. I have found it extremely difficult to accept responsibility for my own thoughts and deeds. Thanks to the tremendous assistance of the Holy Spirit, I have made progress on this huge problem and I am convinced today that overcoming rationalization is a huge factor in the excellent mental health I enjoy today. John 8:32 says, "Then you will know the truth, and the truth will set you free." When we rationalize, we are, of course, denying God's Truth and the results can be devastating.

Later in Genesis, Chapter 4, we find the story of Adam and Eve's sons, Cain and Abel. Both sons offered sacrifices to God. Both boys, I assume, understood God's rules for sacrificing. Abel accepted the rules and offered a sacrifice pleasing to God. Cain, however, rationalized his unpleasing sacrifice by thinking it would be okay to offer fruits of the soil as his offering, instead of what God commanded. When God rejected Cain's offering, Cain became very angry. God asked him why he was angry (as if He didn't know) and reminded him that if he did what was right, he and his offering would be accepted.

Then God made this remarkable statement, which most certainly is still applicable today. "If you do not do what is right, sin is crouching at your door; it desires to have you, but you must master it." (Gen. 4:7) It has gradually dawned on me, through these many years, that my tendency to rationalize is the same as "sin crouching at my door." With the help of the Holy Spirit, I simply must learn to master it. As I look back over my past years, I can now see that rationalization was a big factor in bringing on many, if not all, of the illnesses that I have endured.

Many years ago, one of my church deacons invited me weeks in advance to go deer hunting with him. Now ever since my early childhood days, I have truly loved to hunt and fish. I was really looking forward to this hunting trip in particular. A few days before I was to leave on this scheduled trip, I had gotten off my daily health habits. For several reasons, I wasn't exercising, eating, sleeping, or resting as I should have. And, I had developed the initial symptoms of a cold. My beloved wife saw my condition and she requested I opt out of the hunting trip. Then, she literally begged me not to go because the weather turned very rainy and cold. She knew it was a very bad idea to be out deer hunting in those conditions, especially with my cold symptoms. But, I rationalized, saying God would take care of me. I told her I would dress warmly and I would be careful. Sure enough, after being outside throughout the first day, in the cold and wet weather, looking unsuccessfully for my deer, I became very sick.

I dragged myself home and spent several days in bed with the flu. I was miserable the entire time. My beloved wife never said "I told you so" because she didn't need to say a word. I had learned a very valuable lesson through that experience. It has served me well, even to this day, 33 years later. I fully believe that one of the main reasons I enjoy excellent health today is that I have stopped rationalizing away the truths and conclusions of great health. I have made progress in searching for, finding, believing, and putting into practice God's wonderful truths which He has so generously given to us through His Holy and Written Word. And, I have paid attention to and heeded the "facts" of my body, the weather, and other health indicators and influencers. I believe this awareness and deduction is nothing more than thinking and believing correctly, while refusing to rationalize away the facts.

Keeping Sharp

You know the old expression, "Use it or lose it"? I firmly believe this applies to thinking and using your brain. One way to exercise your brain is to play games. Playing games gives levity and fun to life, and when played with others, can also be a great way to build relationships. I love to play games with my family. Some of these are indoor, thinking-oriented, family card games, like Flinch, Animal Game, Hearts, Rook, Authors, and Go Fish. Other games are car or travel games such as Alphabet, Animal, Vegetable or Mineral; Guess the Name of a famous Person I'm thinking of, etc. I also love other indoor games like chess, checkers, scrabble, cribbage, gin rummy, shuffleboard, bridge, Chinese checkers, and word puzzles that appear in the newspaper like Jumble.

If games aren't your style, try a hobby that requires a life-long journey of learning and discovery. Learn a trade like cooking or woodworking. Become an artist and learn the tools and tricks of the various mediums you use. Learn to write fiction or a screenplay for a movie. Or, go back to school and learn a new mentally challenging discipline. Even if you never use your new found education in a new career, it's good to flex your brain and learn reasoning skills that are applicable to your field of study.

These types of activities are especially important if you have a job that does not require a lot of brain power. I applaud and commend all who take on jobs that require more physical labor than thought. These jobs are necessary to make the world go round, and our economy would plummet without them. But if you have a job like this, you need to find activities to exercise your brain as well as your body. If you are physically fit and also mentally fit, then God can use you for specific and wonderful purposes to accomplish His goals on this earth. All your strengths will become an asset, and you can take great joy in knowing you are being of service to God and mankind.

Finally, I want to conclude that every person, physically fit or not, mentally bright or not, could and should read and/or listen to Scripture daily. As stated in John 1:1 earlier in this chapter, God is the Word, and the Word engages both the mind and spirit. I have come to really appreciate 2 Timothy 3:16-17 which says, "All Scripture is God-breathed and is useful for teaching, rebuking, correcting, and training in righteousness, so that the man of God may be thoroughly equipped for every good work." When you are mentally and spiritually well-fed by a steady diet of Scripture, you are mentally and spiritually ready for every task God has assigned you to do.

Chapter 11
Healthy Thoughts on Politics and Government

"Tell us then, what is your opinion? Is it right to pay taxes to Caesar or not?" [Jesus answered,] show me the coin used for paying the tax." They brought Him a denarius, and He asked them, "Whose portrait is this? And whose inscription?" "Caesar's," they replied. Then He said to them, "Give to Caesar what is Caesar's, and to God what is God's." - Mathew 22:17, 19-21

Also, seek the peace and prosperity of the city to which I have carried you into exile. Pray to the LORD for it, because if it prospers, you too will prosper. - Jeremiah 29:7

Until I was married to Margaret Ann, I was more of a centrist on the political spectrum. I was moderate on all facets of life (politics, religion, life-style, etc.) My motto for years had been "Conservative in Theology and Liberal in Spirit." In the 1950s in Mineral Wells, Texas, one of my church deacons was Chairman of the National Democratic Party. He was close to House Speaker Sam Rayburn, and Campaign Chairman for Lyndon Johnson, when Johnson ran for the U.S. Senate. And, this deacon was very active in Johnson's bid to become President. This deacon and I were close friends and I identified closely with the Democratic Party. At the time, the Democratic Party was quite conservative in Texas. I considered the Democrats to be the Party of the People and the Republicans to be the Party of Big Business.

Margaret Ann grew up in a very strong Republican family and believed each person should be responsible for him or herself. Helping hands from government programs were okay, but not hand-outs. She identified with the Apostle Paul's letter to the Thessalonians, where in 2 Thessalonians 3:10-13 he comes down pretty hard on those who wouldn't work. He said, "For even when we were with you, we gave you this rule: 'If a man will not work, he shall not eat.' We hear that some among you are idle. They are not busy; they are busybodies. Such people we command and urge in the Lord Jesus Christ to settle down and earn the bread they eat. And as for you, brothers, never tire of doing what is right."

With these words, the Apostle Paul strongly encouraged personal responsibility. So, when Margaret Ann's husband left her and their four young children, she refused welfare and went to work for Bank of America. She accepted monthly payments from her ex-husband but no government dictated alimony. When we met in 1974, she and her children had had only one vacation in 12 years and that was a trip to Iowa financed by her parents. They packed seven people in one car for that trip. She simply insisted on living within her budget. She was determined not to go into debt.

Margaret Ann has helped me see that work should always

come before pleasure. She has shown me that accepting responsibility in life and being obedient to the Will of God are our top priorities. I, in turn, have helped her see that it is okay to have some fun in life and also to understand the old saying, "all work and no play makes Jack a dull boy."

So, I began to identify with the Republican Party as the party of hard work, personal responsibility and Biblically conservative values. The Republicans seemed to have convictions and a platform that was more in line with what I had come to believe. Nevertheless, I am not enthused about either of the major parties today and consider myself more of an Independent. I strongly believe in my conservative Christian values and I will not compromise when it comes to sticking with the truths and values taught to me from the Bible, Genesis through Revelation.

American Politics Today

Modern American politics seem to be enamored with life on this earth, as if that is the only thing that counts. Our founding fathers and Presidents of old, on the other hand, always seemed to have an understanding and knowledge that their Creator was watching over them. But today's politicians, in general, seem to have forgotten about the guiding hand of Providence. They have forgotten about spiritual and eternal life and they now legislate on short-sighted thinking. Too often they legislate not out of reverence to the Almighty, but out of deference to special interest groups, or other less principled nations they wish to placate, or out of their own selfish interests. While our American politicians may talk a good game, many don't appear to have our nation's interest at heart. They are rejecting the faith and the practices of our forefathers, many of whom fought (and died) valiantly for our country. Both major parties today have compromised their values in order to accommodate baser values and I think that is very wrong!

In particular, I believe too many politicians have listened far too closely to the gay and abortion agendas. Lobbyists for both agendas have had major influences with both Republicans and Democrats. All of the USA has been affected by them, but California, my home State, seems particularly hard hit.

As of this writing, the health care debate rages on in America. I share the same concerns as *Focus on the Family* and what like-minded political awareness groups share on the subject. I believe a nationalized healthcare program could likely force American taxpayers to pay for abortions. It could force doctors and nurses to violate their consciences by performing abortions. And, State mandated abortions could eradicate many pre-existing state and local ordinances that already are set in place to restrict the abominable practice. This is wrong! I'm also not interested in having my tax dollars, in the form of nationalized health care, go to treating preventable sexually transmitted diseases that are contracted by those who intentionally and deliberately engage in promiscuous behavior that is singled out in both the Old Testament and New Testament (of the Holy Bible) as being contrary to the Perfect Will of our Beloved Creator.

Despite whatever our government does, there is hope. Psalm 42:11 says, "Why are you downcast, O my soul? Why so disturbed within me? Put your hope in God, for I will yet praise Him, my Savior and my God." Here, David confesses his depression and negative attitude and lack of faith and then answers his own questions by saying the answer is having faith in God and being obedient to Him.

Many Americans, Christians included, love to complain and harp about the government. It seems to be our favorite indoor sport. We often feel helpless when our politicians are acting out of order. Our only recourse, it seems, is to complain and get depressed. While exercising our right to free speech is an American practice and appreciated, complaining about our government is not what God wants nor expects from us. The appropriate response is to pray for our government leaders. They have tremendous responsibilities weighing on their shoulders and if the God of the Bible would hear our prayers for them, He might bless and use the politicians, flawed and sinful or not, to affect some righteous change on this planet.

Listen to these classic words from 2 Chronicles 7:14, "If My people, who are called by My name, will humble themselves and pray and seek My face and turn from their wicked ways, then will I hear from heaven and will forgive their sin and will heal their land."

To experience a healing in our land, we need to pray. We need to stop complaining about our President, our senators, our congressmen and governors, and we need to pray for God's mercy, healing and Will to be done over our local, state and national governments. We need to evoke God's blessing on our homes, schools, churches, and cities. And we need to repent. We need to call our governments to repent. We need to ask God to break our hearts with the things that break His heart, and we need to pray that God would give us the political will to address His concerns over the affairs of our country.

We need to pray to God even if the world and our country appear to be worsening. The Book of Revelation suggests difficulty for the end times. And, many Christians believe we are in the end times today. Many Christians believe the world is experiencing a fulfillment of Biblical prophecy, where we are seeing a polarization of the people into salt and light. Jesus says in Matthew 24:6, "You will hear of wars and rumors of wars, but see to it that you are not alarmed. Such things must happen, but the end is still to come." The culmination of history may be inevitable, but still, our hope (and mental and spiritual health) is dependent on putting our faith in the God of the Bible and enjoying His joy and peace regardless of the political climate around us.

Who you are and what your purpose is here on earth are not dependent on the name or party of the President in the White House. World affairs and national policy do not exempt you from praying for your country and political leaders. The presence of world affairs and national policies dictate that you must appeal to the God of the Bible to bring His presence and healing to our land.

Wisdom from the Ages

In addition to God's Holy Scripture, I have been inspired and taught by great political and social thinkers of the past. These men are heroes of mine, defenders and heralds of truth from the past. They call us, who live in the present, to protect and defend our unique and special form of government.

"The budget should be balanced, the Treasury should be refilled, public debt should be reduced, the arrogance of officialdom should be tempered and controlled, and the assistance to foreign lands should be curtailed lest Rome become bankrupt. People must again learn to work, instead of living on public assistance."

- Cicero, 55 BC

"In this situation of this Assembly, groping as it were in the dark to find political truth, and scarce able to distinguish it when presented to us, how is it happened, Sir, that we have not hitherto once thought of humbly applying to the Father of lights to illuminate our understandings? And have we now forgotten that powerful Friend? Or do we imagine that we no longer need His assistance? 'I have lived, Sir, a long time, and the longer I live, the more convincing proofs I see of this truth, that God governs in the affairs of men. And if a sparrow cannot fall to the ground without His notice, is it probable that an empire can rise without His aid? We have been assured, Sir, the sacred writings that `except the Lord build the House they labor in vain that build it.' I firmly believe this, and I also believe without His concurring aid we shall succeed in this partial building no better than the builders of Babel. We shall be divided by our little partial local interests; our projects will be confounded, and we ourselves shall become a reproach and bye word down to future ages. And what is worse, mankind may hereafter from this unfortunate instance, despair of establishing Governments by human wisdom and leave it to chance, war and conquest. I therefore beg leave to move that henceforth prayers imploring the assistance of Heaven and its blessings on our deliberations, be held in this Assembly every morning before we proceed to business."

- Speech to the Constitutional Convention, June 28, 1787 by Ben Franklin

"It is impossible to rightly govern a nation without God and the Bible."

- George Washington, First President of the United States of America

"Our Constitution was made only for a moral and religious people. It is wholly inadequate to the government of any other."

- John Adams, Second President of the United States of America

"We hold these truths to be self evident: that all men are created equal; that they are endowed by their Creator with certain inalienable rights; that among these are life, liberty, and the pursuit of happiness"

- Thomas Jefferson, Declaration of Independence Author and Third President of the United States of America.

"Government should do for people that which they cannot possibly do for themselves – and leave otherwise alone."

- Abraham Lincoln

"In answer to your inquiry, I consider that the chief dangers which confront the coming century will be religion without the Holy Ghost, Christianity without Christ, forgiveness without repentance, salvation without regeneration, politics without God, and heaven without hell."

- General William Booth, Founder of the Salvation Army, spoken about the 20th Century

Personal Responsibility

Lately, it has been the fashion of our government to throw money at our financial, spiritual and physical health problems, wishing they will go away. This idea is foolish. Money is not the answer. We've thrown money at a lot of our troubles and we are no better off today than when we first fell into trouble. What we need is to swallow a large dose of truth and let that truth mobilize us to new action, living life in Truth, by the Truth, for the Truth.

President Thomas Jefferson once said, "Information is the currency of democracy." I'd like to use those words and create a similar saying, "Truth is the currency of good health." Good intentions, untested policies that sound true but really aren't, and well-wishes will not bring you the good health you really need. Now is not the time to take stabs in the dark with our national health. It's time to return to what made our nation great to begin with, and return to the values of the Declaration of Independence and the Bill of Rights.

In today's politically correct world, many politicians, educators and pundits will tell you lots of buzz-words and by-lines to try and give you hope. They will placate you and make you feel better with catch-phrases. But at best, these words are a prelude to willy-nilly, "let's-try-and-see-if-this-will-work" legislation that acts as a mere band-aid to deeper issues. (Frankly, I believe a lot of our issues are just plain sin: acting wrongly.) At worst, this legislation (like welfare) may actually bring you harm and hurt your mental, spiritual, emotional and physical wholeness and healing. At best, it will probably cost the taxpayers a lot of money and may delay or eventually prevent you from gaining your own mental, spiritual, emotional and physical wholeness and well being.

I believe one of our biggest mistakes is the modern day welfare programs. We are missing the mark. There is too much emphasis on sympathy and not enough on empathy. Our government encourages people to go on welfare and stay on welfare. The public is accepting this offer of public assistance. Those who accept welfare think they can do better by being on welfare than by being on their own. As such, they become dependent on the government to simply exist. Many on welfare are not being taught the fundamentals of living responsibly. Instead, our government tends to coddle these people with offers of free this and free that. And today, it seems free money and services from the government are commonplace. Regrettably, voters vote in these politicians and these politicians keep doling out the programs.

In 1960, Democratic President John F. Kennedy said at his inaugural address, "And so, my fellow Americans: ask not what your country can do for you - ask what you can do for your country. My fellow citizens of the world: ask not what America will do for you, but what together we can do for the freedom of man." Now, nearly 50 years after that address, it doesn't seem that most Americans are asking the right questions anymore. They are instead, demanding more and more from our government which seems all too willing to oblige their appetites. Many of today's politicians are far from Thomas Jefferson who said, "the less government the better." I agree.

Unfortunately, our economy has made it difficult to be as prosperous as we once were during the post-World War II period, and even the initial years of the dot com businesses. The news media constantly tells stories about people who say they cannot afford health care, nor make house payments, nor pay rent, or make car payments. They go on and on about the things they cannot afford. It would be interesting to find out the spending patterns of these people, the unfortunate who complain about lack of money. Just what are they are doing with the money they have?

I know of a family on welfare. There's a mother and three children. Each child has a cell phone and they own a computer. The family owns a car, receives free medical care, dental care, and they all eat well. The mother and one daughter are addicted to cigarette smoking. They enjoy many luxuries and yet they are still on welfare, dependent on hand-outs. The mother is able bodied and so is the oldest child. Instead of blindly giving the family free money and free programs, the government should be counseling this family to use their resources more wisely. They should also be helping them look for jobs where they wouldn't have to be on welfare. Government offices should establish programs to wean people away from government assistance and towards self-reliance. They should make these people more independent, more self-reliant, and less dependent on welfare.

Furthermore, our government should not expect more financial resources from the "haves" to satisfy the "have nots." Health care is a privilege, not an entitlement. We need to encourage people to become more responsible with their own health as they grow older. People should be eating right, exercising more and working harder to get out of poverty and into greater independence. If welfare-recipients practice these behaviors in increasing measure, then they can begin to enjoy the blessing of being able to give instead of merely receiving.

How Christians Can Lead

I know times are difficult these days, and my heart goes out to people who have experienced a streak of so-called bad luck. I believe the Church (and not the government) could and should lead the world in providing many of the services our government today tries to provide. If the Church is the "hands and feet" of Christ, I think we could and should be able to provide food, health care, and education more competently than godless government programs. What a witness to the world we, the Church, could be if we would give to those in need and show them a way out of their problems and poverty. If we offer care "in Jesus name" rather than in "Uncle Sam's name," the world will know that Jesus is their provider and not the government.

James 1:27 says, "Religion that God our Father accepts as pure and faultless is this: to look after orphans and widows in their distress and to keep oneself from being polluted by the world." What a witness to the world we, the Church, would be if we took care of widows and orphans properly.

I believe every city should have well stocked food pantries with food donated by our local churches, farms and grocery stores. I'm sure the churches and Christian farmers and Christian grocery store owners could band together in every city to provide for the homeless and hurting. They just need to do it. Leviticus 19:10 says, "Do not go over your vineyard a second time or pick up the grapes that have fallen. Leave them for the poor and the alien. I am the LORD your God."

Think about all the lawyers who do "pro bono" work. This is "free" work they do to help those who cannot afford it. Why can't all the Christian doctors, dentists and service personnel band together and to the same? Provide free care for those in need in our community.

And more importantly, why can't Christian teachers and those who merely care about others, band together and teach basic life skills to those who cannot afford it? This could and should include classes in public and private schools. Everyone should know how to balance a check book, save money, live on a budget, and live a disciplined life. There are some poor out there who do not want to live responsibly, but if government programs are cut off and Church-based, faith-based options are available to them, they will turn to someone who serves them in the name of Christ. Unfortunately, some will never receive help or change their lives, but are we responsible for the ones who will not change? All we can do is say, "We are available if you need help. We'll serve you if you want it." If someone refuses help, what can we do?

Big government is not the solution. Why should hard-working taxpayers pay money into a system that has lots of fat and red-tape to serve people who are unwilling to become hard-working tax payers themselves? Compassion is essential, yes, but not from the government and not with taxpayer money. Politicians should be compassionate as individuals because they are compelled by the love of Christ evidenced in their own lives. Compassion must come from the Church, which reflects the hands and feet of Christ.

When the Church steps up and says, "I will serve Christ by doing anything and everything to serve Christ. I will live sacrificially. I will give until it hurts." Then and only then, will the Church fill a need that Government seems all too anxious to fill today.

I'll close with a story about the Black Death, which occurred between 1348 and 1350 throughout Europe. A pandemic disease was spreading, most likely an outbreak of bubonic plague. The horrible disease killed an estimated 30% - 50% of all Europeans. The amount of devastation this disease brought upon the world was far bigger and more horrible than AIDS and Swine Flu combined. It was estimated that victims would die within 60 – 180 days of contracting the disease. Malnutrition, poverty, disease and hunger, coupled with war, and growing inflation compounded. Many shook their fists at God and asked, "Why aren't you stopping this?" But a few other faithful Christians, went into the areas hardest hit by the plague and served the sick, sealing their own doom. Disease victims sought sanctuary and help in the monasteries, and gave the illness to the monks and friars. These men of God sacrificed their own lives for others.

My prayer is not for bigger government, but for bolder Christians. I pray for revival in our land, where people would turn from their wickedness and selfishness and instead, turn to God for all their needs and sustenance. I pray that God would give meaningful, well-paying work to others and that He would empower people to do their jobs exceedingly well. And, I pray for righteousness to return to our government, where our President and leaders would understand it is by the Grace of God that our nation is preserved.

Chapter 12
Great Financial Health: Handling Your Money God's Way

Give, and it will be given to you. A good measure, pressed down, shaken together and running over, will be poured into your lap. For with the measure you use, it will be measured to you.
- Luke 6:38

No one can serve two masters. Either he will hate the one and love the other, or he will be devoted to the one and despise the other. You cannot serve both God and Money.
- Matthew 6:24

At an early age, my parents wanted to teach me how to handle money. So beginning in 1926, when I was 5, they gave me a weekly allowance of 5 cents. I was able to keep three cents for my personal use and the other two cents were to be given to the Lord. My parents gave me a box of dated and numbered envelopes. One side of the box had envelopes for the local church and the other side of the box had envelopes for missions. Each week, I put one cent in each side and thus learned about sharing my financial blessings with the God of the Bible and His Work here on earth.

Jump ahead to the first week of January 1950. At that time, I began my pastoral ministry at the First Christian Church of Woodson, Texas. I was still in seminary at Texas Christian University in Fort Worth, Texas, so we agreed on a modest salary of $30 per week. My first wife and I decided we would always put our tithe each week into the church where we were serving. We gave our tithe to First Christian Church. Within one month after starting as pastor, the Church Board voted to increase our weekly income to $40 per week. They also built a parsonage next door to the church so my wife and I and our 1-year-old son could have a place to stay when we traveled to Woodson on Friday afternoons. We would stay there until after the Sunday evening church service. This was a tremendous blessing.

In 1965, due to my first wife's inability to cope with being a pastor's wife, our entire family moved back to Mineral Wells, Texas where some of my former church members, plus some community leaders, helped me put together a non-profit Corporation called Palo Pinto Community Service Corporation. We hoped we could qualify for federal funding to fight the War on Poverty. My salary was set at $800 per month, with the understanding that I was not to be paid until we had money in the bank. We sold our home in Tulsa, Oklahoma for a fair profit, so we had a little money to live on for a few weeks. But, with moving expenses and buying a house in Mineral Wells, we needed more money. So I borrowed $2,000 from a local bank. I used up all of our savings in a few months in anticipation of getting funding from the Office of Economic Opportunity (OEO).

Finances were getting rather tight when Sargent Shriver, Head of OEO, came to Texas Christian University in Fort Worth to promote the War on Poverty. I drove to Fort Worth and managed to get in a few personal words with Sargent Shriver, who seemed genuinely interested in what I was doing. In a few weeks, he not only gave us our initial funding (a trial period of 6 months) but he told his staff to give national attention to our ministry in Palo Pinto County. An Associated Press reporter from Dallas called me and he ended up writing a great article, which appeared in newspapers all over the United States in 1966. I eventually paid off the loan at the bank and within a short time was debt free. This corporation today is called Texas Neighborhood Services and it has an annual income of over 40 million dollars. Furthermore, Texas Neighborhood Services represents 11 counties as they continue to fight the War on Poverty.

These three stories above represent God's great faithfulness and goodness to those who put their financial life in His hands. I could not have experienced these enormous blessings in my life if it wasn't for God leading and guiding me throughout my life. I also give enormous credit to my parents, wife Margaret Ann, and family for helping me and encouraging me as well. It's never too late to learn good financial principles and it's never to late to have your friends and family learn too. When they come on board with you and help keep you financially accountable, your path to great financial health is clear and straight. If your family won't help you to be accountable with your finances, find a support group that will help you.

Approaches and Responses to Finances

Some Christian believers seem to love money more than God. They are motivated by greed. They behave no differently than those who reject God for a life of financial gain. They'll even sacrifice their own health to gain another dollar. They are like the people mentioned in this verse: "Whoever loves money never has money enough; whoever loves wealth is never satisfied with his income. This too is meaningless" (Eccles. 5:10).

Other believers are on the complete opposite side of this spectrum. They seem to hate money and confuse this verse, "For the love of money is a root of all kinds of evil. Some people, eager for money, have wandered from the faith and pierced themselves with many griefs" (1 Tim. 6:10). These people are so afraid that money will lead them to evil that they shun it altogether and live hand-to-mouth not knowing where their next meal will come from. They literally beg from others to get their sustenance. For the record, the verse above does not say "Money is the root of all evil," but rather the love of it.

Both of the above reactions to money above are out of order. The appropriate response to money is to serve and love God above all else, to use money as a tool for greater service to God and for greater effectiveness for God's purposes, and finally to support yourself and your family. Understanding your role in the Kingdom of God, obeying God's commandments on how to use money, and daily seeking the guidance of the Holy Spirit will help you understand your role in God's economy.

If you are blessed with understanding numbers and you

are careful with money, perhaps God will use you to make money to bless others. I believe God has blessed many Americans with money and the ability to make money so they can support ministries both domestically and overseas. We should not take God's blessings for granted. The Bible says He can and will remove these blessings if a nation forsakes Him and His Perfect Will.

Other people are not blessed with the ability to make money. For them, money, budgets and spreadsheets are confusing. These people also may simply have a tremendous heart to serve others without compensation. Think of missionaries who take care of the poor in other countries. Even so, every one of us can use our money biblically or unbiblically, and everyone can learn what the Bible has to say about using and handling finances correctly.

Read now about the lifestyle the Apostle Paul had when he was ministering in Thessalonica. "As apostles of Christ we could have been a burden to you, but we were gentle among you, like a mother caring for her little children. We loved you so much that we were delighted to share with you not only the gospel of God but our lives as well, because you had become so dear to us. Surely you remember brothers, our toil and hardship; we *worked night and day* in order not to be a burden to anyone while we preached the gospel of God to you" (1 Thess. 2: 6-9).

A good work ethic, regardless of how much money you make is always appropriate and will always yield some kind of reward. Ecclesiastes 5:19 says, "Moreover, when God gives any man wealth and possessions, and enables him to enjoy them, to accept his lot and be happy in his work—this is a gift of God."

The bottom line is that money is neither good nor bad. It's a commodity that can be used for good or bad. It's a tool, and no matter how much or how little you have of it, it belongs to God. You are its manager.

Tithing

One way you can act biblically with your personal finances is to give 10% or more of what you earn to your local church. This is a practice of giving back to God, and it is called tithing. It's a way to say to God, to yourself and to others, that you recognize the money you earn belongs to the Lord. It's a way to put your faith to the test. And the tithes collected from the whole church body can be used to fund a larger work than you could achieve with your tithe alone. Malachi 3:10 says, "'Bring the whole tithe into the storehouse, that there may be food in My house. Test Me in this,' says the LORD Almighty, 'and see if I will not throw open the floodgates of heaven and pour out so much blessing that you will not have room enough for it.'"

This is an awesome promise. Even before we married, Margaret Ann and I gave our tithes in obedience to God. Around 1936 in her home State of Iowa, Margaret Ann's parents began giving her 30 cents a week allowance, with the strict understanding that 10 cents was for personal spending, 10 cents was for her church, and 10 cents was for savings. (In all actuality then, this was a 33% tithe!) She was given three Calumet Baking Powder cans with her name on each can, marked for spending, church, and savings. Margaret Ann was about three years old when she started getting this allowance. Her sister and brother were older, but each had their own Calumet Baking Powder cans. Margaret Ann has been tithing ever since, and now believes in tithing, 100%, even if it hurts.

And it seemed to hurt her later in life. When Margaret Ann was a single mom with four young children, times were tough. Nevertheless, she still gave her tithe to her local church, and every time she gave she felt a tight pinch in her wallet. (Incidentally, I was a pastor at this church, later in life.) At this time, Margaret Ann had too much month at the end of the money and she had to make a frightful choice one early December. She had to decide if she should give her tithe or buy Christmas gifts for her children. She didn't have enough money to do both. After prayer and reflection, she decided to give the tithe and she told her four children not to expect anything for Christmas. The decision devastated her, but she felt compelled to obey God. Two weeks later, her parents unexpectedly gave her $400 to be used for her family. Her parents were unaware of her financial need, and yet God used them to bless her for her faithfulness. Margaret Ann believes this is a great miracle, an example of God's faithfulness to us when we are faithful to Him.

I tithed as a boy growing up in a pastor's family. Upon reaching college and being on my own, I discontinued tithing and only gave as I felt like it. I acted the same through my four years in the Navy. Once I started singing in the two gospel quartets and making more money than I ever had in my life, I became convicted of the need to tithe. So in 1946, I again started tithing. Furthermore, I began to give offerings to selected Christian ministries. Right or wrong, I felt I needed to makeup for the years I did not tithe. Today Margaret Ann and I believe our tithe should go to our local church and our offerings to other ministries beyond that. We offer financial support to nine other Christian ministries beside our local church.

My wife and I honestly believe the God of the Bible has blessed us for doing this, although we do not do it for the blessings. We do it simply because we believe it is the will of God and we support the Lord's continuing ministry here on earth. We do not consider tithing a legal requirement, although there is much evidence to support it being such. Rather, we do this out of love and respect for God the Father, Son and Holy Spirit and our profound and indescribable appreciation for our salvation, the gift of God's grace.

If you have not tithed, I encourage you to do so. By not tithing you miss out on the blessing from God that could be yours. By not tithing, you also disobey God. If everyone who attended church regularly gave the church 10% of all they earned, the resources the local church would have would be extraordinary. God is calling you to give. Will you heed the call?

Leaps of Faith

If you are feeling really adventurous, you can give above and beyond the tithe. These financial gifts are called offerings, and represent money greater than the 10% given to the local church. Below are some examples of how Margaret Ann and I have been blessed with giving offerings.

Twelve years ago, with help from some Christian friends, I founded Christian Heritage Ministry, Inc. (a.k.a. Old Fashioned Revival Hour). To fund the ministry, we used money gained through sales of cassette tapes of Old

Fashioned Revival Hour Quartet. (All of us in the Quartet, plus pianist Rudy Atwood, waived any royalties.) After several years, the Board decided we needed to get the Old Fashioned Revival Hour back onto the radio, but it took much more money than we had in the bank. So, after much thought and prayer, I decided I would borrow the money to finance the radio ministry from my retirement account.

I honesty believed I would be reimbursed once the radio ministry was re-established. The radio ministry began again and time passed but it looked like I was going to lose it all. At the lowest point, Christian Heritage Ministry, Inc. owed me a large sum of money. It was a large sum of money for Christian Heritage Ministry, Inc. too. Nevertheless, the money was gone and we weren't seeing any of it in return.

I asked the Board Members to join me in claiming Philippians 4:19 in prayer. The promise of Philippians 4:19 is this. "My God will meet all your needs according to His glorious riches in Christ Jesus." We also prayed that God would give us more listeners, more supporters who could give to our ministry. As we stood on that scripture, within two years, I was paid back the full amount I had borrowed. And, God continues to bless this ministry even to this day. We are now on over 150 Radio Stations, and Christian Heritage Ministry, Inc. is in great shape. We're serving the God of the Bible with faith, hope, love, and enthusiasm. We have over 300 of the original Old Fashioned Radio Hour Broadcasts digitally restored and we have about 200 to go. It's very expensive to do this, but God is blessing our efforts.

As you consider how you should use your money, think and pray about taking a leap of faith. 2 Corinthians 9:7 says, "Each man should give what he has decided in his heart to give, not reluctantly or under compulsion, for God loves a cheerful giver." As you think about cheerfully giving, think about Psalm 37:25: "I was young and now I am old, yet I have never seen the righteous forsaken or their children begging bread." In today's uncertain times, God needs people who are radically dedicated to serving Him. He wants you to be open to giving above and beyond your tithe. He wants you to be available. Seek God and ask His Holy Spirit to show you how you can radically and cheerfully give.

Saving, Spending and Investing

Would you like God to say this to you? "Well done, good and faithful servant! You have been faithful with a few things; I will put you in charge of many things. Come and share your Master's happiness" (Matt. 25: 21). You *can* hear this word from God if you create a profit with the talents God has given you. You *will not* hear these words if you take what God has given you and bury it in the ground and don't try to multiply it. If you do that, God is more likely to say to you, "You wicked, lazy servant! You should have put My money on deposit with the bankers, so that when I returned I would have received it back with interest."

God doesn't want us to be afraid of handling money and taking chances with it. Explore investing your money in business ventures or interest bearing accounts. Handling money correctly is a discipline you learn and practice, just like regular exercise or eating right. While some people are hard-wired to be good with money, everyone can learn how to handle their money better. Everyone can learn how to save, spend and invest.

I recommend that you save between 10 and 30 percent of the money you earn. If you put it in an interest bearing account, you are guaranteed to take out more money than you put in. Today's financial markets are crazy and many people lately have lost great sums of money. But there are some funds that are still yielding a profit. Be sure to check with a financial counselor or advisor before risking a large amount of money. Ultimately, the reason for saving and spending money should be that you believe God is guiding you to do it. The best advice for saving money can be found in Proverbs 13:11, "Dishonest money dwindles away, but he who gathers money little by little makes it grow." This is echoed in Proverbs 6:6-9, "Go to the ant, you sluggard; consider its ways and be wise! It has no commander, no overseer or ruler, yet it stores its provisions in summer and gathers its food at harvest."

With regards to spending money, there is one thing I strongly advise against. That is spending more on credit than you can afford. In other words, don't get into debt. The only debt I believe in is a home mortgage (which hopefully will be an asset to you). A small car payment you can afford every month is also acceptable (but paying for it outright is much better). Although there seems to be some new legislation lately that favors the consumer in debt, credit companies don't really care about your debt. In fact, they make it difficult for you to get out of debt. If you are late with a payment or can't pay a monthly minimum, then they stick you with large fines, putting you even deeper in debt. The borrower is certainly servant to the lender.

If you can pay off your debt through a debt roll-up program or secure a settlement with your creditors, I strongly urge you to do so. You may also want to consider credit counseling or a debt elimination program like www.zipdebt.com. When you are free from debt, you are free to pursue the will of God instead of the will of your creditor, who may not have your best interest at heart. If you live under debt, you can still serve God but you may be tied down to a job you don't like in order to fulfill your monthly obligations. When you have a debt, paying it down becomes your #1 priority, like it or not.

I try to live by the principles of this verse, Romans 13:8 "Let no debt remain outstanding, except the continuing debt to love one another, for he who loves his fellowman has fulfilled the law." There is enormous freedom in life when you are debt free. You are free to love God and love one another.

Matthew 25:29-30 warns us to be wise with our saving, spending and investing. "For everyone who has will be given more, and he will have an abundance. Whoever does not have, even what he has will be taken from him." These words encourage us to use money to bring more abundance into the world. It is no use burying or hoarding your money where it is of no use to anyone. Work in such a way that you can afford not only your tithe (and take care of your own needs), but that you can also bless others with the money you are making. If you store up riches for yourself and not for God, you are no different than the rich fool who built large barns to store all his possessions. Suddenly, without warning, the fool had his life taken from him, and was not able to enjoy the possessions he stored up for himself.

Money is a resource to bless yourself and others. It can be converted into tangible goods and services that can offer genuine change in a person's life. When you earn that money through honest, decent, hard work and transform that money into quality commodities for yourself and others, both you and God are pleased. My prayer for you, dear reader, is that God would lead you out of debt, into abundance, so that you are able to love God and love your neighbor as yourself.

Avoid Name It and Claim It Theology

Awhile back, a book called *The Prayer of Jabez* by Bruce Wilkinson became a large hit in the Christian publishing world. The book is based on a Bible verse found in the Bible, 1 Chronicles 4:10, "Jabez cried out to the God of Israel, 'Oh that You would bless me and enlarge my territory! Let Your hand be with me, and keep me from harm so that I will be free from pain.' And God granted his request." Although Wilkinson never intended this book to be lumped in with the name-and-and-claim-it crowd, this book became a symbol for obtaining great blessing from God, just by claiming it.

The primary culprit to name-it-and-claim-it theology is Mark 11:24, "Therefore I tell you, whatever you ask for in prayer, believe that you have received it, and it will be yours." No other verse in the Bible has been used more to justify greed and misapplied faith. Countless people have read this verse out of context and have used it as a rallying cry to demand whatever they want from God.

Name-it-and-claim-it theologians who wield this verse rarely talk about the verses proceeding and following Mark 11:24. Verses 22 and 23 encourage the reader to have faith in God. In verse 25 God tells the reader how to receive forgiveness. Mark 11:24 was never meant to be isolated and hijacked by false prophets who would seek to use it as a tool to extract money out of the desperate and needy. And yet it is still used that way today.

I heard a well-meaning preacher one day (I was visiting the church he served.) claim in his sermon that you would see money in your bank account if you would simply "believe and claim." He actually said if your bank statement showed a zero balance, it would suddenly have whatever figure you "believed and claimed in the precious name of Jesus." Obviously, this is nonsense and a complete misapplication of God's blessing.

When I look carefully at the many things Jesus says, I conclude that this preacher was acting more in line with 2 Corinthians 3:6, "the letter kills but the Spirit gives life." He was claiming Mark 11:24 without truly understanding it in its proper context. He is one of the many unfortunate people who claim Mark 11:24, but do not understand the Spirit behind it. By the way, my bank balance was fine before and after I went into that service. My bank account remains healthy when I daily apply the good principles of financial stewardship taught to me throughout the Bible.

The Sum of the Matter

Through handling money God's way, Margaret Ann and I daily experience God's blessing. He is "opening up the floodgates of heaven" and "pouring out so many blessings that we don't have room for them" (Mal. 3:10). Are these blessings all monetary? No. Many, if not most of these blessings, are intangible gifts such as love, friendship, and a greater awareness of God's presence and care. We experience freedom such as found in 2 Corinthians 3:17-18. "Now the

Lord is the Spirit, and where the Spirit of the Lord is, there is freedom. And we, who with unveiled faces all reflect the Lord's glory, are being transformed into His likeness with ever-increasing glory, which comes from the Lord, who is the Spirit."

One of the greatest riches I experience today is the simple and good things in life. I enjoy all the wonderful creations of God that are on this planet: the earth, water, skies, animals, plants, etc. I also love the heavenly bodies, the planets, and the stars. Observing all these gifts and enjoying their wonders truly makes my life rich.

But, my greatest joy is enjoying the freedom that comes with obedience to God. When God gives me this freedom, I can also enjoy prosperity and blessing from God. I don't feel guilty about it, even when so many others are not experiencing prosperity. I gain pleasure in knowing that I have pleased God. I see His blessing as a byproduct of His pleasure over me. When you know that God is pleased with you, you don't need anything else. Any material, temporary pleasure (like material wealth) is merely a bonus. Let us pray to be like the Apostle Paul when he says in Philippians 4:12, "I know what it is to be in need, and I know what it is to have plenty. I have learned the secret of being content in any and every situation, whether well-fed or hungry, whether living in plenty or in want."

In the next section, ***Living Your Great Health***, I talk about living your life day-to-day with new purpose. In Chapter 13, I'll walk you through understanding God when you experience ill health. I'll help you understand your place as a child of God and why your great health is an important part of blessing not only your life but others. And I'll conclude with a chapter on leaving a legacy of great health. Your life of great health can help the next generation of health seekers! You are an instrument to help others experience great temporal and eternal life!

Living Your Great Health

Chapter 13
When Ill Health Strikes

His disciples asked Him, "Rabbi, who sinned, this man or his parents, that he was born blind?" "Neither this man nor his parents sinned," said Jesus, "but this happened so that the work of God might be displayed in his life." - John 9:2-3

Is any one of you sick? He should call the elders of the church to pray over him and anoint him with oil in the name of the Lord.
- James 5:14

Man was meant to live forever. And back in Old Testament times, when the earth was young, people lived a lot longer than they do today. The first man, Adam, lived 930 years (Gen. 5:5). Noah lived 950 years when he died (Gen. 9:29). And, Abraham lived 175 years (Gen.25:7). People don't live forever anymore, because sin, death and disease were brought into the world through Adam and Eve's sin. With each successive generation since the dawn of man, the world has felt the cumulative effect of the ravages of sin. New pathogens emerge. And, auto-immune diseases arise due to human gene corruption. Natural disasters also wreak havoc on our lives. All these things reduce our life expectancy. Today, the current average life expectancy rate is around 65 years.[1]

Some civilizations in world history only expected to live around 30 to 40 years or so. A large contributing factor to this low life-expectancy rate was high infant mortality rates. Babies were dying off. Even in the first quarter of the 20th Century, back when I was born, it was common for American families to have multiple miscarriages or babies born that didn't live long. Thankfully, modern medicine, more hygienic conditions and better education have all helped reduce infant mortalities both here and abroad. As of this writing, the oldest living person among us now is a Japanese woman who is 114.[2] Each passing generation should have better health care and better access to preventative and restorative health care. Yet, I believe we won't get much older because sin is still in the world. Satan is working overtime to "steal, kill and destroy" (John 10:10).

I believe sickness and death are the direct result of sin in this world. Satan took the form of a serpent and convinced Adam and Eve that they would never die if they ate the forbidden fruit. Instead, they were kicked out of the Garden of Eden. God told the couple that they and their children would "return to dust" (Gen. 3: 19). They were told they would experience death. Sickness and things that lead to our deaths (like diseases) are bound to happen. Last I checked the mortality rate for us humans is 100%. Disease and death are a part of our human experience, but they don't have to define us or limit us. Your spirit and body can experience a great touch of God, even in the face of disease.

How Disease and Death Can Do Good

Let me get this straight from the beginning. God *is not* the author of disease and death. Sickness, death and decay are not a part of God's original plan for earth and its inhabitants. I'll say it again. God *is not* the author of disease and death. God does, however, temporarily allow Satan to bring disease and death into the world because God can use disease and death to teach a lesson to His followers.

Romans 8:28 says, "We know that in *all* things God works for the good of those who love Him, who have been called according to His purpose." If all things can work for our good, then that includes sickness and disease. It is naive to think that God only wants your health and happiness here on earth. Although it may be hard to understand, wholeness and perfect peace are reserved for heaven only. What the God of the Bible desires of you most, during your time here on earth, is your obedience and commitment to Him. And, He'll use anything, including pain and disease, to influence you towards faith in Him. As C.S. Lewis wrote, "Pain is God's megaphone to rouse a deaf world."

Do you remember Job from the Bible? Job was a man, who was "blameless and upright; he feared God and shunned evil" (Job 1:1). If ever there was a man who didn't deserve pain, disease, and calamity, it was Job. Job was a sort of all-star in the faith. He was captain of God's team. He was a leader among men. And, yet, bad things happened to Job. In addition to his livestock and children taken away from him, Job was inflicted with painful sores from head to toe. Job's friends and Job's wife told Job to curse God. But, Job did not. Job said, "Shall we accept good from God, and not trouble?" (Job 2:10). And throughout it all, Job did not sin against God.

Job endured long lectures from his friends, but he remained steadfast in his faith in God. Job prayed for his friends and then the Lord made Job prosperous and well again. The Lord blessed the latter part of Job's life more than the first. (See Job 42:12.) In this case, God used sickness and pain to test Job's faithfulness. Job proved a faithful servant and was in return blessed by God.

Other times, God allows pain and sickness to occur for a limited time, only to heal the disease later. John 9:1-3 says, "As He [Jesus] went along, He saw a man blind from birth. His disciples asked Him, 'Rabbi, who sinned, this man or his parents, that he was born blind?' 'Neither this man nor his parents sinned,' said Jesus, 'but this happened so that the work of God might be displayed in his life.'" Jesus went on to heal this man, and this healing led to a long debate among the Pharisees investigating the healing. The healing also resulted in further teachings by Christ to His disciples about His own divinity. Many great lessons came out of that healing.

Healing or miracles occur so that God can draw attention to Himself. God allows sickness and disease to occur sometimes because He knows that when He does heal it, it will cause a discussion among those who witness (or even hear about) the healing. Healings don't seem to be as common today as they once were, especially in North America. But in regions of the earth where people are less skeptical of divine healing (like Africa and parts of Asia), reports come in almost daily where the healing touch of God is manifested. (If you want to hear reports of what God is doing in the world, I highly recommend you subscribe to news services like AssistNews.net or Missionary International Service News Agency [MISNA].)

One other way that God uses sickness and disease is to *not* heal it. Who hasn't seen a family that has a child with Down Syndrome? Doesn't your heart go out to them? Don't you think, "How courageous!" You are inspired by people with disabilities or people who care for those with disabilities because you realize they are enduring despite setbacks. If you are a Christian, you may already know about Joni Erickson Tada, a quadriplegic who cannot move her arms or legs, and yet she inspires countless people daily with her messages of faith on radio, books and television. God could have healed her, but her disability gives her a platform for ministry.

You may also have heard of Nick Vujicic, a young Australian man who was born without arms or legs. God may never "heal" him, but Nick has a world wide ministry where he speaks about God's faithfulness and authority. Nick's testimony is incredible, and inspires others to faith and belief in Jesus Christ. If Nick wasn't born this way, would he be able to reach and touch as many people as he has? I don't think so. From his website, Nick says, "Psalm 139:17-18 is one of my favorite Scriptures. It says, 'How precious to me are Your thoughts, O God! How vast is the sum of them! Were I to count them, they would outnumber the grains of sand.'" Nick is not looking at what he lacks, but on what God provides. That is inspirational, and it's a lesson we can all learn from. Count your blessings, not your disabilities.

What about healing?

God is a healer, and He still heals today. But He only heals after faith is applied, both in Biblical times and today.

You and/or your friends and family need to intercede and ask God for healing before He will do it. Even if God doesn't heal you or your friend, one thing is certain. If you or your friends and family don't ask God for a healing, He will not give you one. Healing follows faith.

Luke 5:12-16 tells of a leper being cleansed. It reads, "While Jesus was in one of the towns, a man came along who was covered with leprosy. When he saw Jesus, he fell with his face to the ground and begged him, 'Lord, if you are willing, you can make me clean.' Jesus reached out His hand and touched the man. 'I am willing,' He said. 'Be clean!' And immediately the leprosy left him. Then Jesus ordered him, 'Don't tell anyone, but go, show yourself to the priest and offer the sacrifices that Moses commanded for your cleansing, as a testimony to them.' Yet the news about Him spread all the more, so that crowds of people came to hear Him and to be healed of their sicknesses. But Jesus often withdrew to lonely places and prayed."

There are three lessons here to observe. First, the God of the Bible can and will heal us, provided it is His will. It appears to me through Scripture reading and by observing healing today, that God is most interested in giving healing if it will incite faith in Him. This is not something we should try to predict either. I encourage you to not second guess God, if He doesn't bring healing, even if you think a healing would do a lot of good in the world. Isaiah 55:8 says, "'For My thoughts are not your thoughts, neither are your ways My ways,' declares the LORD."

Next, Luke 5:12-16 says we need to request healing and not take it for granted. When we get lazy and assume God will heal us, then we are saying we now know better than God. Know that He is a healer, request your healing, and let Him decide what to do. You may also need to keep praying for healing, even over many years, in order to see it happen. The point is to let God know you believe in His power and sovereignty in prayer, in addition to believing it in your heart.

Lastly, we need to express our appreciation to God for all He does for us. Philippians 4:4 says, "Rejoice in the Lord always. I will say it again: Rejoice!" If you can daily put into practice, believe and live as Psalm 106:1 says, "Praise the LORD. Give thanks to the LORD, for He is good; His love endures forever," this greatly improves the chances that no disease can touch you. You are undefeated and hopefully experiencing a form of great health that few understand or experience. Whether we are healed or not of our infirmities by the God of the Bible, we are to praise Him for all He is and all He does.

I think of the time I was in seminary, 1949, at Texas Christian University. Dr. Roy Snodgrass, Dean of Students, preached a sermon I still remember today, on the need for Christian faith in all circumstances. He had three points. "We need faith because of the facts, faith in spite of the facts, and faith beyond the facts." If the facts are giving you a grim diagnosis, have faith. Faith will give you hope, regardless of what happens to you. If God heals you, you have a testimony. If God doesn't heal you, your endurance and faith in God, despite your troubles is a testimony. If you die because of your disease, you'll be in the presence of the Lord, no longer experiencing pain, and you'll be the envy of all of us who remain on this earth, suffering through this sin-wracked life.

My fervent hope and prayer is that this book will serve

as a source of encouragement to *all* who read it, even the chronically ill. My heart goes out to all who battle pain and/or frequent doctor visits and/or a shortened life expectancy. I do not write this book without thinking of you nor do I write with disregard of the daily struggles you face.

My own Health Struggles

When I first began writing this book, I was suffering from a virus that my medical doctor assured me was not life-threatening. He told me it would disappear in a week or two. Neither he nor I knew how or why I got the virus, but we both know it was for real and it was no picnic while it lasted. Actually, I believe it was an attack from Satan, since he does not want people to read this book. If this is true, I consider it a real compliment and I wish to praise and thank God for His confidence in me.

While I suffered through the virus, I did not write anything for three weeks. During those three weeks, I suffered like I had never experienced before and hope to never experience again. I am convinced, now more than ever, that my illness was an attack from Satan to try and scare me off and discourage me from continuing with the project.

This can happen, and if you are doing front-lines ministry, it's important to appeal to God for protection. Satan doesn't attack people who are already defeated, but those who are willing to step out in faith in obedience to God. Satan stands ever ready to attack, like a prowling lion.

Let's go back to my illness. Though it was only a temporary virus, it was so devastating that I lost my will to live and I suffered deep depression. I was like 2 Corinthians

1:8 where Paul says, "We do not want you to be uninformed, brothers, about the hardships we suffered in the province of Asia. We were under great pressure, far beyond our ability to endure, so that we despaired even of life." My illness was so terrifying that I wrote down two prayer requests for my beloved wife. I asked her to first pray that God would restore my desire and will to live. Secondly, I asked her to pray that God would restore the joy of my salvation and remove my despair. Margaret Ann's prayers were constant, sincere, compassionate, fervent, emotional, zealous, earnest, faithful and Scriptural. Neither of us gave up on the fact that God was listening and would answer in His own time and in His own way.

Three weeks later, I was nearly entirely healed of this terrible illness. I'm ready to get back into the harness of carrying out our Lord's daily assignments. Did my physical health temporarily suffer? Yes. Great health doesn't necessarily mean continual, excellent physical health. Great health is knowing Who your protector, provider, healer and friend is, even as you are suffering poor health. It's a win-win situation!

God Promises to Care For You

Now is a good time to address God's promises, since they are such an integral part of everything I am trying to say in this book, and because they played such a huge role in bringing me successfully through this recent illness. I've also included some commentary in parenthesis to tell you how these Scriptures have blessed me.

"Those who sow in tears will reap with songs of joy."
- Psalm 126:5
(There is hope at the end of every illness for those who believe.)

"The LORD Himself goes before you and will be with you; He will never leave you nor forsake you. Do not be afraid; do not be discouraged."
- Deuteronomy 31:8
(During illness and at all times, God is with us.)

"God is our refuge and strength, an ever-present help in trouble."
- Psalm 46:1
(This verse needs no explanation. God is always there!)

"Give thanks to the LORD, for He is good; His love endures forever."
- 1 Chronicles 16:34
(Another clear verse. With God's love sticking with you forever, you can endure it all.)

Looking Within

When I encounter any problem whatsoever related to my health, I look at myself and I look at what I have done recently to contribute to the problem. My first thought is *not* to schedule an appointment with my medical doctor and expect him to give me my good health back. Usually, I discover the problem I'm experiencing is a result of something I ate or drank or did (like playing golf on a cold, wet day when I felt a cold coming on). In other words, I find the problem is my fault. I diagnose how or why I got into poor health, and if I use common sense,

I can usually figure out a way to get better.

If you overeat, use tobacco or alcohol, or otherwise perform risky acts of behavior, look at yourself if you are experiencing a health problem. If there is some behavior you can modify to prevent your health problem, then change it. Don't blame your friends, your doctor, or today's society for your preventable health problems. Blame yourself. Repent. And change. After all, God wants you and me to enjoy great health as much as possible. And if you are practicing poor health habits, you are denying Him the opportunity to bless you.

For many years, I have maintained that I am my own best "doctor." I know what is best for my own body. No one can possibly know my body as I well as I know it, since I have lived in it and with it for over 88 years. My present medical doctor is a very capable man and he is excellent at what he does. He knows bodies, but he doesn't know my body like I know my body. If I am unable to handle any personal physical problem that arises, I do not hesitate to contact him for his input, evaluation, recommendation and treatment. But in the final analysis, the responsibility for my health belongs to me, not him. It is my body and I'm ultimately responsible what happens with it and to it.

Bizarre Treatments

I believe that all good gifts are from God, even medical gifts that seem odd or out of place. In 1976, I had cancer cells on my face. My medical doctor in Fresno recommended that I go to a skin cancer specialist. This man, Dr. Swineheart, looked at my face and ears and said I needed a treatment of Efudex. He said applying Efudex on my skin would halt the cancer and pull it out of my system. For seven days morning and night, I covered my face, ears, eyebrows, and neck (front and back) with Efudex cream. I looked as if I had leprosy. My face was white and flaky. I looked like a horrifying freak. Remarkably, I believe it drew out the cancer! For a period of time, I said, "Will I ever look normal again?" Seven days later, it was smoother than it had been in a long, long time. It was amazing. I was free from skin blemishes and today I'm cancer-free.

I've also relied on naturopathic doctors who rely on natural methods or remedies for fixing my illnesses. This is a holistic approach that advocates a minimal amount of surgery or drugs. Many times, their services have worked and have gotten me well again. Again, whatever is helpful is a gift from God.

In 2 Kings, Chapter 5, the author talks about a man named Naaman, the commander of the army of the king of Aram. Naaman was told about a healer, the prophet of the Lord, Elisha. Elisha sent a messenger to Naaman and said, "Go, wash yourself seven times in the Jordan, and your flesh will be restored and you will be cleansed." Naaman didn't like this idea. He thought it was silly. He wanted Elisha to attend to him personally and touch him. Elisha refused to do this, however. He did not visit Naaman and he did not touch him. After a little more convincing, Naaman went down to the Jordan River, and he dipped himself into it seven times. There, Naaman found his healing. Even though you may hem and haw over what sounds like an odd treatment, be willing to try something new, like Naaman, who was willing to try something unconventional.

I believe God can use anyone or anything to bring

a healing. God can use medical doctors, chiropractors, and naturopathic doctors, etc. He can also use herbs, diet, and treatments found outside of the popular medical establishment to treat diseases. Nobody has all the answers. All who would hope to bring healing and treatment to others need to listen to each other and work together. A treatment that works should be celebrated and recommended. If it has worked for someone, it is worth exploring. If God is telling you to seek a treatment somewhere other than a hospital or a clinic operated by an M.D., you should obey God's call.

In Conclusion

Years ago, a man jokingly told me of a new sulfa pill. I asked him what it did. He told me it would help me lose weight. I bit on the joke and asked the man the name of the pill. He laughed and said, "Sulfa Denial." There is no shortcut to gaining great health. It requires doing all the things I have talked about so far in this book. It requires discipline.

It also requires discipline and will power to seek God in prayer for healing and/or strength when you are facing illness. It's not easy living here on earth. But, the Holy Spirit can give you the power to live well and the power to pray and the power to face treatments valiantly.

A beautiful painting exists by Nathan Greene entitled "Chief of the Medical Staff." The painting depicts Christ standing in a high-tech modern operating room, guiding the hand of the surgeon who is cutting into the body of a patient. This artwork is a great painting to study for all those who are facing their own surgery or medical procedure. It's a fantastic reminder that we are always in God's care, even when we are most vulnerable. Whether we are healed, or enduring a long illness, we are in good hands; we are in the hands of the Chief of the Medical Staff.

Footnotes

1. http//en.wikipedia.org/wiki/Life_expectancy.
2. http://en.wikipedia.org/wiki/Oldest_people.

Chapter 14
You Have a Purpose

The LORD will fulfill His purpose for me; Your love, O LORD, endures forever— do not abandon the works of Your hands. - Psalm 138:8

Being confident of this, that He Who began a good work in you will carry it on to completion until the day of Christ Jesus. - Philippians 1:6

An old parable tells of a farmer getting ready to plow for corn in his cornfield. Just as he was about to put his hand to the plow, he looked up into the sky and witnessed a life changing experience. There, across the blue expanse, he saw three huge letters, "GPC." Being a dedicated Christian, he quickly knew what he had to do. He let go of the plow and decided he must "Go Preach Christ." Surely, that was what the good Lord was telling him to do. The farmer ran to the farmhouse and told his wife and children that they would be selling the farm and starting a new church in town.

Many years later, after completely failing as a preacher, the farmer died and entered the Pearly Gates. The farmer was pleased that he had obeyed God all these years but he was curious to know why he was such a failure. There at the gate, Saint Peter told the farmer, "Your misread the letters, my dear brother. The letters meant 'Go Plow Corn', not 'Go preach Christ.'" Amazed at his own folly, the farmer-turned-pastor shook his head.

This funny little tale is a sermon illustration that I gave when I wanted to talk about purpose. The lesson, of course, is to be sure of your calling. God has hard-wired each and every one of us with different skills and different interests. Although we each perform different functions, we are all part of the same body, the Bride of Christ. We are all working for a singular purpose: to serve the God of the Bible and to proclaim His Lordship over all the earth.

A Lesson On Purpose

Let's look at the verses from Romans 12:1-2. "Therefore, I urge you, brothers, in view of God's mercy, to offer your bodies as living sacrifices, holy and pleasing to God—this is your spiritual act of worship. Do not conform any longer to the pattern of this world, but be transformed by the renewing of your mind. Then you will be able to test and approve what God's will is—His good, pleasing and perfect will."

When you say the words, "Not my will but Yours be done," you offer yourself as a living sacrifice to God. When you say and believe that statement, you put God's desires and Will before your own. God loves this kind of worship above all else. (Many people merely think of worship as singing. It's actually all about living your life in devotion to God.) You renew your mind by continually worshipping and praising God, and by spending time in His Holy word. You are able to understand God's Heart and Will toward humanity when you read how He has related to humans in the Bible. Since "Jesus Christ is the same yesterday and today and forever,"

(Heb. 13:8) you can expect that He will call you in the same manner He has called others in the past. You can discern how He acts and speaks today, based on how He has acted and spoken in Biblical times.

Therefore, if you immerse yourself in the Bible, you can learn to discern the difference between His will and the world's will. You will be able to test and approve what the God of the Bible wants you to do. (He'll never ask you to do or say something contrary to what He has already said or done in Scripture.) It is very important to daily spend time in God's word so you can monitor your life and your life activities against what He would like you to do. Knowing how to please God and live with a sense of purpose is dependent on understanding how God acts and speaks toward His believers – both in Biblical times and today.

Romans 12:3 further explains the meaning of your purpose. "For by the grace given Me I say to every one of you: Do not think of yourself more highly than you ought, but rather think of yourself with sober judgment, in accordance with the measure of faith God has given you." Humility and honesty are crucial if you are to fulfill your calling in life. If you think too highly of yourself, you'll encounter troubles when you experience stresses for which you are not prepared. If you think too lowly of yourself, you'll miss the blessing that could be yours by *not* stepping into the position God has assigned you. I believe God has a calling and plan for everybody, and sometimes this calling is for noble purposes and sometimes it is for more humble purposes, but because you (and I) are called to any position by the God of the Bible, it is a privilege and an honor to serve in that capacity.

Let's continue reading from Romans 12. Here are verses four, five and six. "Just as each of us has one body with many members, and these members do not all have the same function, so in Christ we who are many form one body, and each member belongs to all the others. We have different gifts, according to the grace given us." The Apostle Paul compares the Church to a human body. We are all part of a single person (the Bride of Christ), but individually we each have a distinct purpose. The eye is separate from the brain and the brain is separate from the hand and the hand is separate from the foot. Each of these separate body parts serves a distinct purpose. The question is: Which part of the body are you? What part do you play?

Romans 12:7 suggests distinct and different roles you may play in service to the God of the Bible. "If a man's gift is prophesying, let him use it in proportion to his faith. If it is serving, let him serve; if it is teaching, let him teach; if it is encouraging, let him encourage; if it is contributing to the needs of others, let him give generously; if it is leadership, let him govern diligently; if it is showing mercy, let him do it cheerfully." Whatever our calling may be, each of us is to fully use our gifts, talents and purposes.

Stepping outside your Comfort Zone

Do you know what your purpose is? Do you know your calling? Are you a prophet, a servant, an encourager, a leader, or someone who shows mercy? Perhaps you have a special skill or talent that you can offer God. If you *do know* your purpose and calling, you are blessed. If you *do not know* your purpose and calling, you may have difficulty in life. Many people flounder for years before knowing what God has asked them to do.

There may be a time when God asks you to step outside of your comfort zones to fulfill a very special purpose. He doesn't necessarily consult with your present abilities, but rather He has hope in your future possibilities. He may see something in you that you have yet to see in yourself. You may feel very awkward and strange if God asks you to do something unusual; you might even feel like He is making a mistake. Even so, if by prayer you discover He is asking you to do something you have never done, I suggest you obey. If you disobey, the results can be tragic.

Look at the Old Testament prophet Jonah. God asked Jonah to "'Go to the great city of Nineveh and preach against it, because its wickedness has come up before Me.' But Jonah ran away from the LORD and headed for Tarshish. He went down to Joppa, where he found a ship bound for that port. After paying the fare, he went aboard and sailed for Tarshish to flee from the LORD" (Jon. 1:2-3). On board, the sea grew restless and the boat was tossed about. Jonah 1:15-17 tells the rest of the story. "Then they [the sailors] took Jonah and threw him overboard, and the raging sea grew calm. At this the men greatly feared the LORD, and they offered a sacrifice to the LORD and made vows to Him. But the LORD provided a great fish to swallow Jonah, and Jonah was inside the fish three days and three nights." If you disobey God and His calling, He may cause a calamity to happen to you. He could cause a great fish to swallow you whole!

From inside the great fish, Jonah prayed these words to God, "Those who cling to worthless idols forfeit the grace that could be theirs" (Jon. 2:8). If you disobey God's direct orders, you are clinging to a worthless idol. You are saying to God, "My way is better than Your way. I'm going to serve the god of my own appetites and desires instead of You, the God of the Bible." This decision is dangerous territory to tread because not only might you be swallowed by a great fish (just one example, of course), but you also might not get a second chance to obey God and follow His calling.

Thankfully, Jonah got a second chance. "And the LORD commanded the fish, and it vomited Jonah onto dry land. Then the word of the LORD came to Jonah a second time: 'Go to the great city of Nineveh and proclaim to it the message I give you.' Jonah obeyed the word of the LORD and went to Nineveh." (Jon. 2:10 – Jon. 3:1-3) As a result of obeying God, the people of Ninevah repented of their sins. They fasted for 40 days, and the king of Ninevah declared "Let everyone call urgently on God. Let them give up their evil ways and their violence" (Jon. 3: 8). Your obedience can cause a city of 120,000 people to repent. You are important in the scheme of God's plans.

When God calls you, you should be like Samuel instead of Jonah. The young Samuel, who was serving the prophet Eli, lay down to sleep. God called Samuel but Samuel did not yet know the Lord nor the Lord's voice. Samuel rushed to Eli to inquire if he had called him. Eli did not. "So Eli told Samuel, 'Go and lie down,' and if He calls you, say, 'Speak, LORD, for your servant is listening.' So Samuel went and lay down in his place. The LORD came and stood there, calling as at the other times, 'Samuel! Samuel!' Then Samuel said, 'Speak, LORD, for Your servant is listening.'" And the LORD spoke to Samuel and told him to send a message of warning to Eli. Samuel obeyed and talked to Eli. Eli listened. And, God continued to speak to Samuel. Samuel listened and was used mightily throughout his life.

This type of calling by God to one of His followers is also heard in Isaiah 6:8-9. "Then I heard a voice of the Lord saying, 'Whom shall I send? And who will be willing to go for us?' And I said, 'Here am I. Send me!'"

If you obey the God of the Bible and get into a habit

of reading and studying His word and hearing His voice, you can become a powerful instrument in His hands. God is looking for someone who will listen and obey. Will that person be you?

Many of us, as we age into our 30s, 40s and beyond, merely survive. We work at a job we don't like, to live unhappy lives. It is what Henry David Thoreau says in his book *Walden*, "The mass of men lead lives of quiet desperation." The God of the Bible does not want you to live a life of "quiet desperation." The God of the Bible wants to give you an "abundant life" (John 10:10). And, an "abundant life" stands in stark contrast to a life of "quiet desperation."

If you obey the call of God in your life, your spiritual, physical, emotional, and mental health will have a great chance of flourishing. Your life will definitely *not* be "quietly desperate." If you obey the call of God in your life, you can live happily and effectively through the power of the Holy Spirit. Your efforts can be tremendously fulfilling. If you are serving God with a joyful heart in your work, you will never work a day in your life without the joy of the Lord. All your efforts, even if some of your efforts are stressful, can be counted as all joy.

What is Your calling?

One way to discern your calling is to look at these three indicators: your interests, your opportunities, and Holy Scripture. When these three align, it's a good chance you can find your purpose and calling. Let's break down each one of these elements one by one. Your interests, of course, are what you like to do. You may love to serve people and give them acts of service. You might like to speak, or write, or organize, or clean. You are fulfilled by doing for others what they cannot or will not do for themselves. The God of the Bible gave these interests to you. You are excited about doing these kinds of things because this is how He hard-wired you. Your interests are God's way of telling you if you are a hand, an eye, a foot, a mouth, or some other body part in the Body of Christ.

Your opportunities are the offerings that life presents to you. Your church may have a ministry fair where opportunities of service may be presented to you. If you want to serve God at the local church, you can attend a ministry fair and see what opportunities are available. Other opportunities include community volunteer jobs as well as actual money-paying jobs. You can serve God by serving others in a wide variety of ways. Have fun trying different opportunities for service. If one job doesn't work out, that's okay. You can try another area of service until you find a good fit.

Finally, look at Scripture. As I said before, the God of the Bible will never ask you to do something that He doesn't approve of in Scripture. He'll never ask you to be a liar, a murderer, a thief, or an adulterer. These are prohibited by the Ten Commandments, and these Commandments still apply today. The God of the Bible *does* approve of teaching, healing, serving, helping, and preaching among many other things. These are all Biblically acceptable avenues of ministry. Of course, God could supersede your interests and call you to go to a place like Nineveh. But, He more often plants interests in your heart, gives you opportunities to practice your interests and then confirms it by Scripture.

My Calling

My call to preach was a gradual call that started after I joined the Goose Creek Quartet of the Little Country Church of Hollywood, and Charles E. Fuller's Old Fashioned Revival Hour Quartet. When I sang with these quartets, I heard dozens and dozens of sermons over a four year period. Our Quartets would be invited to sing at a church service, a youth rally, an evangelistic meeting, etc. and then after we sang, we'd sit down and hear the pastor or evangelist preach. I heard sermons Sunday mornings, Sunday afternoons, Sunday evenings, and during the week, for four years in a row! Throughout this time, God gradually spoke to my heart, mind and soul and told me this is what He wanted me to do.

Three years into the four year period when our quartets were most active, I got to the point where I had to make a decision about this call to preach and pastor. I had to obey the call or I had to leave the Quartets. I was driving down Hollywood Boulevard in my Packard one day when I got this overwhelming urge to dedicate my life to full-time Christian service as a pastor and preacher. I had to make a decision.

I thought of the old James Lowell hymn, "Once to every man and nation, comes the moment to decide." He wrote the hymn in 1845 and the lyrics read, "Once to every man and nation, comes the moment to decide, In the strife of truth with falsehood, for the good or evil side; Some great cause, some great decision, offering each the bloom or blight, And the choice goes by forever, 'twixt that darkness and that light."

Born in Cambridge, Massachusetts, in 1819, James Russell Lowell graduated from Harvard in 1838. After obtaining his law degree, he became an ardent champion of abolition. In 1876, President Hayes appointed Lowell as Minister to the Court of Spain, and in 1880 the President transferred him to Great Britain. Over the years, the influential and eloquent James Russell Lowell was in great demand as a public speaker. (As a man dedicated to serving God, he stood before rulers and authorities.)

Originally written as a protest poem, "Once to every man and nation," first appeared in print on December 11, 1845, in the *Boston Courier*. The lyrics voiced Lowell's protest against the war with Mexico over the territory of Texas. Lowell feared the acquisition of a new territory would only enlarge the area of slavery in the United States. Eventually, music was added and the poem of protest became a hymn of challenge. The initial challenge was this, "Will the U.S. annex Texas, or will it not?"

Now, it was my time to face the challenge God was giving me. Would I annex the Lord's call on my life, or would I refuse and separate myself from Him? Would I brush aside His call and continue to sing with the Quartets? Or would I take a leap of faith? I decided "Yes" to God. I decided to become a pastor. In 1947, I pulled over on Hollywood Boulevard and said, "I'll do it, God. You show me the way." Shortly after that prayer, Dr. Charles E. Fuller took me aside and said, "Say Dick. Why don't you enroll in my first class at Fuller Theological Seminary?"

There, in front of such evangelical greats as Dr. Charles E. Fuller and Dr. Harold Ockenga (co-founder of Fuller Theological Seminary), Dr. Carl F. H. Henry, Dr. Edward Carnell, Dr. Harold Lindsell, Dr. Everett Harrison, Dr. Wilbur Smith, and Dr. Gleason Archer; I learned great truths of Scripture, as well as skills and tools to become an effective pastor and preacher. My classmates included, among others, Bill Bright (founder of Campus Crusade for Christ), Dr. Ralph Winter (noted Missiologist and Founder of the U.S. Center for World Missions), Dr. Gary Demarest (who became a dynamic Presbyterian pastor/preacher and married the daughter of Dr. Louie H. Evans, senior pastor at First Presbyterian Church of Hollywood, from 1941-1953),

Bill Gencarella (who helped me get the Old Fashioned Revival Hour back on radio), Dr. Albert Strong (a missionary in Ethiopia and dynamic Presbyterian minister in Oregon), Dr. Charles B. and Alice Carlston (distinguished Christian educators), Robert Gerry (well known missionary in Japan), John Winston (Belgian, leader and great evangelist in Europe), and Dr. Daniel P. Fuller (son of Charles E. Fuller).

As I reflect on my years at Fuller, I also think of Proverbs 22:29 which reads, "Do you see a man diligent and skillful in his business? He will stand before kings; he will not stand before obscure men." By saying "Yes" to the calling I was given, the God of the Bible placed me in the presence of great men. These men taught me well, and they gave me the best education possible. I, in turn, went on to befriend, know or work with other great men of the faith including Charles C. Chapman (Founder of Chapman University, the first mayor of Fullerton, California, and a relative of John Chapman, the legendary "Johnny Appleseed"), Dan and Ruth Fuller (Dan is the only child of Charles E. and Grace Fuller), M. Howard Fagan (pastor of the large Wilshire Boulevard Christian Church for many years in Hollywood), and J. Vernon McGhee (host of *Thru the Bible* radio program).

I also got to know Charles Templeton (Canadian cartoonist, evangelist, politician, newspaper editor, etc.), Bob Pierce (a great Youth For Christ Leader and Founder of international charity World Vision), Billy Graham (internationally renowned evangelist), Cliff Barrows (longtime music and program director for the Billy Graham Evangelistic Association), Hoagy Carmichael (American composer, pianist, singer, actor, and bandleader), Bob Hope (American comedian, actor and United Service Organizations [USO] entertainer), E. Stanley Jones (Methodist Christian missionary and theologian to India), Richard Mouw (current

President at Fuller Theological Seminary), Russell Spitler (a well-known Assembly of God preacher, writer, scholar, professor, and administrator), and James and Shirley Dobson (founders of *Focus on the Family*).

I don't wish to brag about meeting or knowing these people. I only list them to tell you about them to let you know that by obeying the call of the Holy Spirit, and by becoming a disciple of the God of the Bible, the likelihood is high that you will serve amongst the best of the best. Being a devoted disciple is not a calling to obscurity. It is a calling to partner with other like minded people who have whole-heartedly abandoned themselves to doing the Will of the God of the Bible.

I'd like to paraphrase a quote from Bill Bright, my fellow classmate and founder of Campus Crusade for Christ, "The world has yet to see what a man fully devoted to Christ can do." Despite the fact that he and I and you are sinners, I believe Bill Bright was a man fully devoted to Christ. Today, Campus Crusade for Christ has penetrated over 190 nations of the world with the Gospel. The organization has led countless lives to the saving knowledge of Jesus Christ, through the work of the *Jesus* film and one-on-one discipleship. Your future is wide open with possibilities if you become fully alive to the God of the Bible, and fully obey the call that He has placed on your life.

Being a pastor hasn't always been easy, but it has always been fulfilling and challenging. One final thing I want to add here about answering the call of God is the idea of being "always available." If you look at the life of Jesus, He was always interrupted by people. He would be going somewhere and then He'd be stopped by someone in need. God wants you to be ready to serve at a moment's notice. 2 Timothy 4:2 says, "Preach the Word; be prepared in season and out of season; correct, rebuke and encourage—with great patience and careful instruction." The lesson here is to be prepared at any time and in any situation to receive a message or an assignment from your Creator.

Here are other Biblical examples of God appearing quickly before others. In Luke 1, Zechariah was going about his daily routine when an angel appeared with the news that Elizabeth would conceive and give birth to John the Baptist. In Luke 2, the shepherds were doing their everyday shepherd work when an angel appeared with the news about the birth of Jesus. It is not our option to decide how and when God will show up and call us to this or that. It is our job to be ready for instant direction, should God decide to do a quick work. It is the openness and availability to be used by God, for God, at any time and in any situation. It is what I call, "Interruptability," and it is a trait that all mature Christians should have.

In Conclusion

Do you remember this children's hymn? "I am a promise. I am a possibility. I am a promise with a capital 'P.' I am a great big bundle of potentiality, and I am learnin' to hear God's voice. And I am tryin' to make the right choice; I am a promise to be anything God wants me to be. I can go anywhere that He wants me to go. I can be anything He wants me to be. I can climb the high mountains, I can cross the wide sea. I'm a great big promise you see!"

I cannot break down the purpose for your life any simpler than that. It's all about hearing God's voice and then being all He wants you to be. God also spells it out simply in Old Testament days with Deuteronomy 30:15-16. The passage reads, "See, I set before you today life and prosperity, death and destruction. For I command you today to love the LORD your God, to walk in His ways, and to keep His commands, decrees and laws; then you will live and increase, and the LORD your God will bless you in the land you are entering to possess." When you obey God, God will "bless you in the land you are entering to possess." When you heed His calling, your life improves.

Deuteronomy 30:19-20 goes on to say, "This day I call heaven and earth as witnesses against you that I have set before you life and death, blessings and curses. Now choose life, so that you and your children may live and that you may love the LORD your God, listen to His voice, and hold fast to Him. For the LORD is your life, and He will give you many years in the land He swore to give to your fathers, Abraham, Isaac and Jacob." In these excellent verses, God gives us choices. We can choose great health (life) or poor health (death). The choice is ours. God's purpose for you is great health, but it's your choice whether you will accept it or not. If you choose life by obedience and faith in God, your spiritual, physical, emotional and mental health will stand the best chance to be great.

Chapter 15
Leaving a Legacy of Great Health

For you know that it was not with perishable things such as silver or gold that you were redeemed from the empty way of life handed down to you from your forefathers, but with the precious blood of Christ, a lamb without blemish or defect.

- 1 Peter 1:18-19

Train a child in the way he should go, and when he is old he will not turn from it.

- Proverbs 22:6

One of the best things about enjoying great health as the years go by is the opportunity to pass along my knowledge and example to younger generations. My great health is a gift, and it's a gift that needs to be shared. I believe I have the privilege and the responsibility to pass along to others the wisdom I have gained and the example I have become due to God's grace. I have been blessed, and so I believe I should bless others too. It's the "pay it forward" principle.

My favorite way to leave a legacy of great health is to start with my own family. As far back as I can remember, my family has always meant a great deal to me. (And, of course, they continue to be a personal treasure.) I enjoy giving them my time and attention, as well as my wisdom and insight. Showing them the way to great health helps me gain great health. Third John verse 4 perhaps best explains how I feel about the relationship I have between my excellent health and my wonderful family. It reads: "I have no greater joy than to hear that my children are walking in the truth."

Margaret Ann and I together have been blessed with nine wonderful children (and their wonderful spouses), plus thirty-two wonderful grandchildren, and twenty wonderful great-grandchildren. I could write an entire book about the blessings they have been to us. Their achievements and success stories delight us. And, we relish the love and respect they have given us, from the day they were born to the day of this writing.

An old saying among writers is this, "You never finish a book, you just abandon it." There is so much I could include here on my family, but I'll save it for a later book. Perhaps in my next book or two, I'll tell you more about my individual family members and I'll also tell you their stories. My family gives me so much joy, and it's hard for me to imagine enjoying excellent health apart from joy. This joy (and all joys) is from the Lord. As Nehemiah 8:10 says, "The joy of the LORD is your strength." Joy, family and health just seem to go together, hand-in-hand.

As we sow Truth into the lives of our family members, we trust that they, in turn, will eventually bless others too with the Truth they have learned, if they haven't already. This is the essence of leaving a legacy of health: living and modeling a healthy life and helping others to achieve it too.

It's all about teaching great spiritual, physical, mental and emotional truths to others. 2 Corinthians 9:6 says, "Remember this: Whoever sows sparingly will also reap sparingly, and whoever sows generously will also reap generously." We hope to sow generously into the lives of the next generation to leave a legacy of great health.

Let's look now at a sad story that tells a different tale. A reliable source told me of a very fine, up-right man and a loyal citizen of our beloved country, who became an attorney, and later a judge. He was very intelligent and capable, but his education and experiences took him away from what he was once taught. As a child, he was taught that Jesus was His Lord and Savior. As an adult, he still claimed to be a believer, but he didn't live like one. He forgot the instruction of his youth, and his faith became stagnant. He did not live like he had an active, important relationship with the God of the Bible. Unfortunately, this man came down with a series of illnesses and eventually passed away. During the last few weeks of his life on earth, he confided in a friend that he was going from one doctor to the next, suffering from one ailment after another. He was very dejected and depressed, and yet he was unwilling to return to the Christian faith that once dominated his life. He spent thousands of dollars trying to regain his health, but he never recovered it. Furthermore, during his adult life up to the point of his death, he was quite consumed with his own self interests. Apparently, he never shared Christ with anyone else, and he certainly didn't model great health for anybody. In my opinion, this man died a tragic figure.

Leaving a legacy of great health is more than doing good deeds that will help the next generation. It's a Biblical mandate to disciple others with the Truth and Understanding of the God of the Bible. And as you live a life demonstrating the God of the Bible to others in word and deed, you'll help keep the powers of evil at bay. The aforementioned attorney/judge, who died after a series of illnesses, is a sad example of what the enemy (Satan) can do to a man not committed to living by and through the Truth. He exchanged the Truth for a lie and he had little to no sense of spiritual purpose. Satan struck him when he was down and kept him down. As such, he left no legacy of great health.

When you are filled with the power of the Holy Spirit, you can fight against Satan and his schemes to ruin you and your loved ones. I agree with the prayer of Ephesians 3:16 which says, "I pray that out of His [God's] glorious riches He may strengthen you with power through His Spirit in your inner being." When you have the power of the Holy Spirit working within you, your life (and death) can be a testimony to the goodness and greatness of God, as well as be a shield to Satan's plans to steal, kill and destroy.

When you are living a life of active faith, sharing with others the goodness of God in your life, and praying for the redemptive plan of Salvation through Christ to come to those you love who do not know Christ, God shows up and you can actively sense His presence. When you get serious with God, He gets serious with you. He shows up like a daily silent partner guiding you and instructing you in the way you should go. The more obedient you are to God, the more He shows up in your inner being, being your Leader, Counselor and Friend. When you can sense the power of God, it's easy to tap into His power to help others. It's an exciting, palpable feeling. I agree with the Apostle Paul's prayer in Philemon 1:6, "I pray that you may be active in sharing your faith, so that you will have a full understanding of every good thing we have in Christ." When you share your faith and your lives with others, you can begin to understand the goodness of God.

The famous evangelist, Dwight L. Moody, trying to explain the mystery behind the enormous power of his sermons, stated that the more he did for God, the more power he seemed to have. I can identify that assessment. When I do God's will, living life His way, I feel God's presence and power.

The Mantle

A mantle is something that covers, envelops, or conceals.[1] A mantle also means a blessing that you give to another, such as your family members and/or your younger friends. It means you wish to impart to them the same favor, power, energy, and purpose that God has given you. A mantle is most effective when given actively, as in the form of a prayer or blessing.

Look at Genesis 27. When Isaac (son of Abraham) was old, he wanted to bless his son Esau with a prayer. Esau was the first-born son and had the right to experience the best blessing, or greatest mantle, from his father. But Isaac's wife Rebekah, wanted the younger son, Jacob, to receive the first blessing. So she came up with an elaborate scheme involving slaughtering young goats, and Jacob wearing goat fur on his arms, just so that the aged, blind Isaac wouldn't know the difference between his sons and would instead give Jacob, not Esau, the first blessing.

This is the text of the first blessing that Isaac gave his

second son Jacob, from Genesis 27:28-29, "May God give you of heaven's dew and of earth's richness— an abundance of grain and new wine. May nations serve you and peoples bow down to you. Be lord over your brothers, and may the sons of your mother bow down to you. May those who curse you be cursed and those who bless you be blessed." When Esau returned from hunting, he realized he had been tricked by his younger brother Jacob. Esau rushed to his father and demanded that his father, Isaac, give him a blessing as well. Isaac relented and eventually gave Esau a blessing, but it was not the kind of blessing Esau wanted. Basically the blessing was more like a warning or a curse. It said Esau would live far away from Jacob and be subservient to Jacob.

Thankfully, blessings no longer come prioritized. Blessings can be given again and again to multiple people. There is no limit on giving blessings and passing mantles to others. And, you don't have to wait until you are near death to pass a mantle down to the next generation. I suggest you pray blessings over the youth in your life regardless of your age or health condition. When you pray over your youth, you set an example of faith and let them know you care. Furthermore, you let the youth know that you believe in the power of prayer. If God begins to work in the lives of the young people you pray for, then they'll become more and more convinced of the goodness and power of God.

After my father passed away, when I was only 12, I sensed the same power and strength in me that I saw in him. As a new orphan (so to speak), I felt the Lord's comfort and assurance and encouragement. I began to experience the same kind of blessing that Jacob experienced after Isaac passed down a blessing to Jacob, and not Esau. I have taken on my father's "mantle," his charge, his legacy and this mantle helped me tremendously. I don't believe my father's spirit is visiting me (like a ghost), but I do believe God's Holy Spirit is assisting me in my Christian walk, the same way He assisted my earthly father when my earthly father was living here on this earth.

If you don't have God-fearing parents, or didn't have God-fearing parents, you may be tempted to disregard your current calling. You may feel like you have a deficient mantle. You might feel like you'll be no different than your less-than-perfect Dad or Mom. Indeed, many people who struggle with life discover they share the same struggles that their fathers and mothers experienced. That's sad. I believe the power of the Holy Spirit can break bad mantles. If you had a bad father or mother and if you struggle with the same sins as he or she, then I suggest you find the Godliest man or woman you know and ask him or her to pray a blessing over you. Ask this Godly man or woman to *keep praying* a blessing over you. See if he or she will intercede for you before the God of the Bible. If an elder in your life commits to pray for you, your steadfast sins stand a great chance to be broken and overcome by the power of the Holy Spirit.

I also urge you that if you already have a great relationship with the God of the Bible, then you should mentor, counsel and pray over younger men and women who are growing (and/or struggling) in the faith. Our younger men and ladies need the prayers and blessing of our older men and ladies. It's Biblical, it's healthy and it helps create such a tremendous sense of God's protection and care.

Other Ways to Leave a Legacy

One way you can lengthen your reach in touching the lives of others is to create media products that can communicate the blessings and Truths you want to pass along. This book is an example of a media message that hopefully will reach many people and will help encourage many people to live a life of great mental, physical, emotional and spiritual health. Sometimes these media opportunities come without even trying. Check out this e-mail I recently received from Dr. David Bundy, Associate Provost at Fuller Theological Seminary.

"Dear Dick: We would like to include the story of your ministry (and that of your father) in the Archives at Fuller Theological Seminary. One of the goals of the David Allan Hubbard Library is to document the ministries and lives of people who have been associated with Fuller Theological Seminary. Your (our) ministries have had a huge impact upon Christianity around the world for the last fifty years. We want scholars to be able to access this story!"

"These personal archival collections may contain a wide variety of materials depending on the arena of your ministry. For example, many will contain correspondence, published and unpublished writings and lectures, sermons (manuscript, tapes, video), sermon research files, church bulletins, photos, résumé, biographical and autobiographical material, bibliography, research notes, syllabi, teaching materials, family history, documentation for professional participation in educational institutions and the Church, audio and video documents, and annotated books. This will include material from one's entire professional and educational career. One cannot give too much! And, we do not need the only copies of materials. If a family member wants a copy or the original, the other will work in the archives. As well, we allow family members to make copies of documents of their relative as stipulated by the donor. So, let's keep talking… and let's preserve your story!"

You can imagine how honored and thrilled I was to receive this e-mail and I will comply with their request as much as possible. I hope people 5, 10, 30 or more years from now will read the materials I submit and learn how they can obtain great health. Furthermore, with the excellent help of some treasured Christian friends, I have resurrected the Old Fashioned Radio Hour broadcasts, making them available to a whole new generation of listeners. The songs, lyrics and music we sang way back when still minister today. These broadcasts, which include hymns sung by our Gospel Quartet, plus the OFRH Choir, can still encourage and give hope to listeners today.

Earlier in the chapter, I told you about how I enjoy sowing Truth into the lives of my family. Family get-togethers, which happen quite often for one reason or another, are just a little taste of what heaven must be like, in my humble opinion. We also like to have family reunions and while there, hold family golf tournaments. One tournament occurs each year the day after Thanksgiving during our Annual Family Reunion at Twain Harte, California which is a mountain community near Yosemite National Park. There, 30 to 50 of our immediate family members gather together in one or two big houses.

This Annual Reunion originally started in 1974 (right after I married Margaret Ann) when we invited our nine children, plus their families, to be our guests at Hume Lake Christian Camp in the Sierra Nevada Mountains for Friday thru Sunday after Thanksgiving. (We call it Family Camp by Hume Lake.) We had 15 absolutely wonderful family reunions at Hume Lake when we then all decided to hold our reunions at Thanksgiving time in Twain Harte instead. All of us enjoy these reunions but I believe it means the most to our grandchildren and great-grandchildren. And I absolutely adore spending time with my grandchildren and great-grandchildren. I'm able to love and guide each one on matters of great spiritual, physical, emotional and mental health. For me, this time is like heaven-on-earth and we plan to continue this tradition as long as possible.

No matter how large or small your family is, I advise you to meet with them all at least once a year. At these family reunion events, you can practice the instruction of Proverbs 27:17, "As iron sharpens iron, so one man sharpens another." At family reunions and other family gatherings, you can sharpen your youth to be as healthy and effective for the God of the Bible as possible. If you have no family or are estranged from your family, I recommend you find a family you can plug into. Your church is a great place to start. As you invest into the lives of children and people younger than you, you can show them your true value. They will come to accept you as a treasured friend.

An Abundant Life

This book is coming to an end, but I hope you can see what great health means to me. Great health is a lifestyle of faith in God, and service to others. When you operate with humility on bended knees in service to your King the God of the Bible, and operate out of the strength of the Holy Spirit in service to others, encouraging them and loving them with the love of the Lord, your health stands the best chance of being great.

As you can see, I look at the word "health" as a very inclusive and comprehensive word. The best synonym I can think of is the word "life." When Jesus promised me an "abundant life (John 10:10)," I believe He was promising me "excellent health." I am convinced that God is blessing me with great health partly because I am committed to Truth. I'm committed to seeking Truth, to accepting Truth, to doing my best to live the Truth, to exposing Untruths, and to the best of my ability, to understand and fight Satan who is living a lie and is the father of all lies.

I always give total honor, glory, credit, and praise to God the Father, Son, and Holy Spirit for Who and What They are and for all They have done. (They are what I have been calling the God of the Bible.) I enjoy what They are doing, and will continue to do, in and through my mind, body, heart, and soul. I believe God, when He calls Himself a jealous God, and I believe that He wants to be #1 in my life. I pledge allegiance to Him, ahead of every other relationship and every situation. Because "God is love" (1 John 4:8), His love spills out into my life onto others. I can give a legacy of great health because God has filled up my spirit so much that it spills out in goodness toward others. I am living proof of Luke 6:38, "Give, and it will be given to you. A good measure, pressed down, shaken together and running over, will be poured into your lap. For with the measure you use, it will be measured to you." God has given me so much, and I wish to thank Him by giving to others the same measure of love and favor that He has given to me.

So, we have reached a turning point in the book. "We have reached the end of the beginning," (word originally spoken by Winston Churchill who said it after England reached an important milestone during World War II). It is an end because we are near the end of the book. It is a beginning because today is the first day of the rest of your life. How will you now live? Filled with "life," or filled with yourself?

My life has been less than perfect. The good Lord knows I have committed many, many sins. But my heart, since age 9, has always been for God, and He has rewarded me with tremendous life lessons and by-and-large great health. I laugh at myself, enjoy my family reunions, and keep in constant touch with family members, especially with my five children, my four step-children, and their spouses. I love and enjoy my body (the temple of the Holy Spirit) given to me by God, and I listen to and obey the Holy Spirit as much as I understand Him. (I believe He gives me direct messages for living.) I learn from my mistakes, live a structured life, and constantly praise God for bringing me through hundreds of extremely difficult situations (some of which were life-threatening). God has seen me through my first marriage and He is leading me through my wonderful second marriage with Margaret Ann.

My prayer for you (and me) is that when we pass away and see our Maker face to face, He will say to you and me, "Well done, good and faithful servant" (Matt. 25:21). If we can live lives pleasing to Him, having done our all for God and His kingdom, we can stand rest assured that we have done our best. Our lives will have been spent in a worthy cause and our legacy will, hopefully, speak to generations after we have gone.

Another Bible verse that encourages me is Acts 20:24, "However, I consider my life worth nothing to me, if only I may finish the race and complete the task the Lord Jesus has given me—the task of testifying to the gospel of God's grace." My final prayer for you and me is that we would leave this earth having finished the assignment God has given us to do. No life can be spent more wonderfully and more gloriously than in devotion and service to his or her Maker.

I don't know how many years I have left on this earth, but I know Who gives life to my years – my Creator and Savior, the God of the Bible. I'd like to leave you with a blessing. May I pray this prayer over you? "Dear Lord Heavenly Father, I pray You would bless my readers with great spiritual, mental, emotional and physical health. Bless them with this health by first blessing them with Your presence. Let them know of Your Glory, Majesty, Power, Strength, and Peace. Lead them by Your Holy Spirit to closer fellowship with You. Call them to Your purposes, and show them how to leave a legacy of faith and great health. Heal them when they are ill, if it is Your Will, but more importantly, show them You are with them when they are in the middle of troubles. Protect them from temptation and deliver them from evil. Let the words of their mouths and the meditations of their hearts be pleasing in Your sight. Bless them in every way, in Jesus' Name, Amen."

I'll conclude with one final brief prayer from one of my most favorite pastors and preachers, noted American clergyman, Phillips Brooks. "Do not pray for easy lives; pray to be stronger people. Do not pray for tasks equal to your powers; pray for power equal to your tasks." God bless you dear reader. I hope we can meet someday and praise God together for what He has done in each of our lives.

Footnotes:
1. http://dictionary.reference.com/browse/mantle?db=luna.

Chapter 16
How You Can Begin to Enjoy Great Eternal Health

For God so loved the world that He gave His one and only Son, that whoever believes in Him shall not perish but have eternal life. For God did not send His Son into the world to condemn the world, but to save the world through Him.
- John 3:16-17

That if you confess with your mouth, "Jesus is Lord," and believe in your heart that God raised Him from the dead, you will be saved. For it is with your heart that you believe and are justified, and it is with your mouth that you confess and are saved. - Romans 10:9-10

The God of the Bible loves you and wants to spend eternity with you. He wants you to enjoy an active, growing, dynamic relationship with Him. If you haven't yet started your life of faith in the God of the Bible, it can begin today. The God of the Bible wants to give you great eternal health. He is your Creator and is jealous for your company.

If you reject the call of the Holy Spirit to have fellowship with Him, He has no choice but to refuse you entrance to Heaven. Those who reject their Creator face an eternity separated from His presence in Hell. (And contrary to what you might think, you won't be enjoying good times with your buddies in Hell. It's all about eternal torment.) The choice is yours. Whom will you serve and where will you spend eternity?

To escape the fires and torments of Hell and to enjoy great eternal health with your Creator, as well as enjoy fellowship with all those who have similarly chosen to believe in the God of the Bible, you must believe and confess.

You must believe (or understand) that you have been living life your own way, trying to do it without Him, the God of the Bible. Living your life, your way, without the guidance and fellowship of the Holy Spirit is living a life of sin. Sin isn't just doing "bad things." Those bad things are bad because you do them separate from faith in the God of the Bible. You could just as easily do "good things" but if you are doing them for your own pleasure and glory, and not for the glory of the God of the Bible, than you are still in sin. So, it is important to recognize you are a sinner and repent (change). Luke 13:5 says "But unless you repent, you too will all perish."

Secondly, you need to believe that the God of the Bible loves you and wishes to forgive you of your sins and be the Lord and Savior of your life. 2 Timothy 2:2-5 says, "This is good, and pleases God our Savior, Who wants all men to be saved and to come to a knowledge of the truth. For there is one God and one mediator between God and men, the man Christ Jesus." If you are not sure of the authority and goodness of the God of the Bible, review John 3:16-17 and Romans 10:9-10. Ask the Holy Spirit to show you who He is and how He has authority over your life.

Now, it is time to confess your sins and ask Jesus to be Lord and Savior of your life. When you confess with your mouth that Jesus is Lord and believe in your heart that God raised Him from the dead, you will be saved. You are saved when you recognize and declare the divinity of Christ and accept His free gift of salvation.

Salvation may be that easy, but Jesus really wants your complete devotion. And this requires daily dying to self and living for Him through His power. Jesus said to the first disciples, "Come, follow Me" (Matt. 4:19). He says the same words to all who would be His disciples today. After salvation, your new life in Christ just begins.

Following Jesus is a lifetime adventure of faith, hope, love, joy, peace, and health. Your life and health won't necessarily be perfect and without difficulty, but it will be better because the God of the Bible will be with you, leading and guiding you. Even if you suffer from life-long, chronic illness, your health and life will be better because you'll have power, love, and fellowship with your Creator. And, you'll also have fellowship with those who have also put their faith in Him.

Will troubles, struggles and sorrows come? Inevitably, they will. God doesn't promise to take away your problems, but He does promise to be with you in the midst of them giving you life and health in this life and in the life to come. As you fellowship and learn from the God of the Bible, you'll live a life of eternal discovery, constant companionship, and powerful purpose.

Encouraging Scriptures found in *Feeling Great at 88*

Note: All Scriptures listed below come from the New International Version of the Bible.

So God created man in His own image, in the image of God He created him; male and female He created them.
- Genesis 1:27

God is not a man, that He should lie, nor a son of man, that He should change His mind. Does He speak and then not act? Does He promise and not fulfill? - Numbers 23:19

The Spirit of the LORD will come upon you in power, and you will prophesy with them; and you will be changed into a different person. - 1 Samuel 10:6

He will yet fill your mouth with laughter and your lips with shouts of joy. - Job 8:21

Taste and see that the LORD is good; blessed is the man who takes refuge in Him. - Psalm 34:8

God is our refuge and strength, an ever-present help in trouble. Therefore we will not fear, though the earth give way and the mountains fall into the heart of the sea, though its waters roar and foam and the mountains quake with their surging. - Psalm 46:1-2

Teach me your way, O LORD, and I will walk in Your truth; give me an undivided heart, that I may fear Your name.
- Psalm 86:11

Trust in the LORD with all your heart and lean not on your own understanding; in all your ways acknowledge Him, and He will make your paths straight. - Proverbs 3:5-6

The sluggard craves and gets nothing, but the desires of the diligent are fully satisfied.
- Proverbs 13:4

A cheerful heart is good medicine, but a crushed spirit dries up the bones. - Proverbs 17:22

"For I know the plans I have for you," declares the Lord, "plans to prosper you and not to harm you, plans to give you hope and a future." - Jeremiah 29:11

...."Not by might, nor by power, but by My Spirit," says the Lord Almighty. - Zechariah 4:6

So do not worry, saying, "What shall we eat" or "What shall we drink?" or "What shall we wear?" For the pagans run after all these things, and your Heavenly Father knows that you need them. - Matthew 6:31-32

But seek first His kingdom and His righteousness, and all these things will be given to you as well. Therefore, do not worry about tomorrow for tomorrow will worry about itself. Each day has enough trouble of its own. - Matthew 6:33-34

Therefore I tell you, whatever you ask for in prayer, believe that you have received it, and it will be yours. - Mark 11:24

Consider the ravens: They do not sow or reap, they have no storeroom or barn; yet God feeds them. And how much more valuable you are than birds! - Luke 12:24

He [Jesus] got up and rebuked the wind and the raging waters; the storm subsided, and all was calm. - Luke 8:24b

Then Jesus declared, "I am the bread of life. He who comes to Me will never go hungry, and he who believes in Me will never be thirsty. - John 6:35

The Spirit gives life; the flesh counts for nothing. The words I have spoken to you are spirit and they are life. - John 6:63

The thief comes only to steal and kill and destroy; I have come that they may have life, and have it to the full. - John 10:10

Jesus said to her (Martha), "I am the resurrection and the life. He who believes in Me will live, even though he dies; and whoever lives and believes in Me will never die. Do you believe this?" - John 11:25-26

I [Jesus] will ask the Father and He will give you another Counselor to be with you forever. - John 14:16

Peace I leave with you; My peace I give you. I do not give to you as the world gives. Do not let your hearts be troubled and do not be afraid. - John 14:27

I [Jesus] have told you these things, so that in Me you may have peace. In this world you will have trouble. But take heart! I have overcome the world. - John 16:33

'For in Him we live and move and have our being.' As some of your own poets have said, 'We are His offspring.'
- Acts 17:28

And we know that in all things God works for the good of those who love Him, who have been called according to His purpose. - Romans 8:28

But the fruit of the Spirit is love, joy, peace, patience, kindness, goodness, faithfulness, gentleness and self-control. Against such things there is no law. - Galatians 5:22-23

Being confident of this, that He who began a good work in you will carry it on to completion until the day of Christ Jesus. - Philippians 1:6

Rejoice in the Lord always. I will say it again: Rejoice! Let your gentleness be evident to all. The Lord is near. Do not be anxious about anything, but in everything, by prayer and petition, with thanksgiving, present your requests to God. And the peace of God, which transcends all understanding, will guard your hearts and your minds in Christ Jesus.
- Philippians 4:4-7

I can do everything through Him (Christ) Who gives me strength. - Philippians 4:13

And my God will meet <u>all</u> your needs according to His glorious riches in Christ Jesus. - Philippians 4:19

Give thanks in all circumstances, for this is God's will for you in Christ Jesus. - 1 Thessalonians 5:18

For the word of God is living and active. Sharper than any double-edged sword, it penetrates even to dividing soul and spirit, joints and marrow; it judges the thoughts and attitudes of the heart. Nothing in all creation is hidden from God's sight. Everything is uncovered and laid bare before the eyes of Him to whom we must give account.
- Hebrews 4:12-13

Without faith it is impossible to please God, because anyone who comes to Him must believe that He exists and that He rewards those who earnestly seek Him. - Hebrews 11:6

Perseverance must finish its work so that you may be mature and complete, not lacking anything. - James 1:4

Humble yourselves, therefore, under God's mighty hand, that He may lift you up in due time. Cast all your anxiety on Him because He cares for you. - 1 Peter 5:6-7

Whoever does not love does not know God, because God is love. - 1 John 4:8

Here I am! I stand at the door and knock. If anyone hears My voice and opens the door, I will come in and eat with him, and he with Me. - Revelation 3:20

Some of Dick Brown's Lifetime Expressions:

- Anything worth doing at all is worth doing well
- Always tell the truth and then you won't need to worry about what you have said
- Always remember we reap what we sow
- The best time to do something is NOW!
- Understanding a problem is 90% of the solution
- One step at a time and one day at a time
- Better to do something poorly than to do nothing well
- I have learned and profited more from my mistakes and failures than from my victories and successes
- Better to light one candle than to curse the darkness
- Don't air your dirty linen in public
- When God gives me an assignment, He gives me the wherewithal to successfully complete that assignment
- Early to bed, early to rise, makes a man healthy, wealthy and wise (Benjamin Franklin)
- This, too, shall pass

- Learn to forgive and forget
- Resist Satan and he will flee
- Keep your head down and eye on the ball (Golfer's Prayer)
- Keep on going and never give up
- Better late than never
- Only one life, 'twill soon be past; only what's done for Christ will last
- Jesus Christ! The same yesterday, today, and forever!!

The Nicene Creed in Modern Language

We believe in one God,
the Father, the Almighty,
maker of heaven and earth,
of all that is, seen and unseen.

We believe in one Lord, Jesus Christ,
the only son of God,
eternally begotten of the Father,
God from God, Light from Light,
true God from true God,
begotten, not made,
of one being with the Father.
Through him all things were made.

For us and for our salvation
he came down from heaven:
by the power of the Holy Spirit
he became incarnate from the Virgin Mary,
and was made man.
For our sake he was crucified under Pontius Pilate;
he suffered death and was buried.
On the third day he rose again
in accordance with the Scriptures;
he ascended into heaven
and is seated at the right hand of the Father.
He will come again in glory
to judge the living and the dead,
and his kingdom will have no end.

We believe in the Holy Spirit, the Lord, the giver of life,
who proceeds from the Father [and the Son].
With the Father and the Son
he is worshipped and glorified.
He has spoken through the Prophets.

We believe in one holy catholic and apostolic Church.
We acknowledge one baptism for the forgiveness of sins.
We look for the resurrection of the dead,
and the life of the world to come.

AMEN